INTERACTIVE REASONING IN THE PRACTICE OF OCCUPATIONAL THERAPY

INTERACTIVE REASONING IN THE PRACTICE OF OCCUPATIONAL THERAPY

SHARAN L. SCHWARTZBERG

Tufts University
Boston School of Occupational Therapy

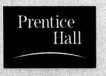

Prentice
Hall

Upper Saddle River, New Jersey 07458

Library of Congress Cataloging-in-Publication Data

Schwartzberg, Sharan L.
    Interactive reasoning in the practice of occupational therapy / Sharan L. Schwartzberg.
       p. cm.
    Includes bibliographical references and index.
    ISBN 0-13-013826-6 (pbk.)
       1. Occupational therapy. 2. Occupational therapy—Philosophy. 3. Medical logic. I.
    Title.

RM735 .S29 2002
615.8'515—dc21

                                                                    2001040039

Publisher: Julie Alexander
Senior Acquisitions Editor: Mark Cohen
Assistant Editor: Melissa Kerian
Marketing Manager: David Hough
Managing Production Editor: Patrick Walsh
Production Editor: Trish Finley/Clarinda Publication Services
Production Liaison: Mary Treacy
Director of Manufacturing and Production: Bruce Johnson
Manufacturing Buyer: Patrick Brown
Senior Design Coordinator: Maria Guglielmo-Walsh
Photography: Sarah Brezinsky
Product Information Manager: Rachele Triano
Composition: The Clarinda Company
Printing and Binding: Courier Westford, Inc.
Cover Design: James Foster-Turner

Notice: The authors and the publisher of this volume have taken care that the information and technical recommendations contained herein are based on research and expert consultation, and are accurate and compatible with the standards generally accepted at the time of publication. Nevertheless, as new information becomes available, changes in clinical and technical practices become necessary. The reader is advised to carefully consult manufacturers' instructions and information material for all supplies and equipment before use, and to consult with a health care professional as necessary. This advice is especially important when using new supplies or equipment for clinical purposes. The authors and publisher disclaim all responsibility for any liability, loss, injury, or damage incurred as a consequence, directly or indirectly, of the use and application of any of the contents of this volume.

Pearson Education LTD.
Pearson Education Australia PTY, Limited
Pearson Education Singapore, Pte. Ltd
Pearson Education North Asia Ltd
Pearson Education Canada, Ltd.
Pearson Educación de Mexico, S.A. de C.V.
Pearson Education—Japan
Pearson Education Malaysia, Pte. Ltd
Pearson Education, Upper Saddle River, New Jersey

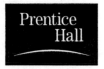

10 9 8 7 6 5 4 3 2 1
ISBN: 0-13-013826-6

BRIEF CONTENTS

CONTENTS

Contents

FOREWORD

I Saw a Bald Eagle Fly

I was driving north on Route 20 to visit the Program in Occupational Therapy at the University of South Dakota on February 22. After leaving Omaha, the landscape bottoms out—quite literally—into a flat and wide riverbottom, bordered on the east by the ancient glacier dust Loess Hills bluffs and bordered on the west by rolling hills that meet the Missouri River. This is an expansive landscape that allows one to wander far and wide in the Big Sky country. About sixty miles north of the city of Omaha, two Native American reservations, the Omaha and Winnebago Nations of northeastern Nebraska, cover the land.

While driving and contemplating this book, I saw a bald eagle flying overhead.

Perhaps it is due to the cross-cultural experience of working with the Omaha and Winnebago Nations over the past five years. Or, perhaps it was just the majestic site of a hunting eagle. Or, perhaps it is the influence of students teaching me about animal spirits through the past years. For whatever reason, I felt the soaring eagle crossing my path at this moment to be totem or animal guide for the foreword of this book.

And not to my surprise, in the world of shamanism, or working with animal spirits, the wisdom of the bald eagle symbolizes everything I wanted to say about this book! I could address the incredible strengths of this text from an academic's perspective. The book is well grounded in primary references. The book is incredibly well researched, etc. But I would rather tell you about this book from a feeling level.

The bald eagle's spirit provides the knowledge of magic, of the illumination of spirit and healing. The bald eagle's spirit pertains to the intuitive and creative spirit and the ability to see the overall pattern. What better description of aspects of interactive reasoning in occupational therapy could there be?

In *Interactive Reasoning in the Practice of Occupational Therapy* by Sharan Schwartzberg, we see the characteristics of the totem of the bald eagle. The work is courageous and possesses wisdom and keen sight into foundations of interactive reasoning in occupational therapy. Issues that continually arise in class discussion with students are directly and profoundly addressed in this text. In fact, my only regret is that this book did not come out sooner for use in occupational therapy education. Certainly, however, it will be a required text in my class next year.

This is not an easy book to read. It has great power and content, which require diligent effort to digest and use. The effort is worthwhile, however, since after working through the material one can rise above the material to see the spiritual or essential nature of interactive reasoning in occupational therapy. The bald eagle's wisdom would identify it as grace achieved through knowledge and the hard work from reading this book.

I saw an eagle fly while driving to the University of South Dakota. I felt a bald eagle fly while reading Dr. Schwartzberg's book *Interactive Reasoning in the Practice of Occupational Therapy.*

It was an honor to be asked to write this foreword, and I hope dignity and grace, the spirits of the bald eagle, become attached to this seminal work.

Charlotte Brasic Royeen
School of Pharmacy and
Allied Health Professions
Creighton University

PREFACE

$\mathcal{M}$y interest in interactive reasoning began after hearing about the Clinical Reasoning Study initiated by Maureen Fleming and Cheryl Mattingly in 1986 (Fleming & Mattingly, 1994; Mattingly & Gillette, 1991). In collaboration with several of my colleagues at Tufts University and University Hospital, Maureen and Cheryl sought to describe the practice of occupational therapists.

Fleming and Mattingly (1994) found that therapists used four modes of reasoning for different purposes. They labeled them procedural reasoning, interactive reasoning, conditional reasoning, and narrative reasoning. Fleming and Mattingly defined the modes of reasoning as follows:

- **Procedural Reasoning.** "Procedural reasoning is used when therapists think about the person's physical ailments and what procedures might possibly alleviate them or remediate the person's functional performance problems" (p.17).

- **Interactive Reasoning.** "Interactive reasoning is used to help the therapist to interact with and better understand the person. Interactive reasoning takes place during face-to-face encounters between the therapist and patient. It is the form of reasoning that therapists employ when they want to better understand the patient as a person. There are many reasons why a therapist might want to know the person better. The therapist might want to know how the person feels about the treatment at the moment; or what the patient is like as a person, either out of sheer interest or . . . to more finely tailor the treatment to his or her specific needs or preferences. Further, the therapist may be interested in this person . . . to better understand the experience of the disability from the person's own point of view" (p. 17).

- **Conditional Reasoning.** "Conditional reasoning, a complex form of social reasoning, is used to help the patient in the difficult process of reconstructing a life that is now permanently changed by injury or disease" (p. 17).

- **Narrative Reasoning.** Narrative reasoning is "making sense of the illness experience" (p. 18) through telling stories that evince a narrative reasoning process.

From Fleming and Mattingly's work, Maureen and I, along with the faculty at the Boston School of Occupational Therapy at Tufts University, developed in 1986 the first curriculum of its kind based on clinical reasoning. This master's degree curriculum has continued to be refined over the past fifteen years. The research derived from Fleming and Mattingly's work is discussed in this textbook and widely applied to the education and practice of occupational therapists worldwide.

The research on clinical reasoning in occupational therapy has continued to this day. This research, along with the author's study of occupational therapists' interactive reasoning, forms the empirical base of the book. Strong evidence persists that supports the original findings of Mattingly and Fleming's work as originally reported in their 1994 textbook on clinical reasoning in occupational therapy. Early on, these authors (1994) recognized that interactive reasoning was highly complex and that it is guided by knowledge of one's own feelings. They wisely recognized that this self-knowledge could be used to understand and even change the feelings of others. Mattingly and Fleming stated, "Careful monitoring and interpretation of one's own and one's clients' behavior must be guided by a particular kind of knowledge and a particular kind of reasoning, which is complex, sophisticated, and essential to therapeutic practice" (p. 196).

This book is intended to unravel the complexity of interactive reasoning in occupational therapy. It is based upon the belief that practice is a composite of philosophy, theory, and empirical data. With this in mind, I decided to structure the book into three sections. The first part comprises three chapters that describe the interactive reasoning practice of occupational therapy.

In chapter 1, The Philosophy, I attempt to answer a preliminary question: What are the founding philosophical and theoretical ideas that underpin interactions in occupational therapy? I looked to the literature in occupational therapy and my own education to select the works of philosophers, psychologists, and occupational therapists described in this chapter. In chapter 2, The Borrowed Practice, I explain the ideas of other professionals from which occupational therapists borrow techniques and theory. Chapter 3, The Occupational Therapy Practice, is central to the book. I believe that the only authentic way to describe interactive reasoning is to ask therapists about their practice and beliefs. This follows the tradition of Mattingly and Fleming's work. Chapter 3 also serves as a point of reference from which my ideas could be evaluated and validated and the contents of the book could be revised in this first edition.

In June of 1999, with the support of a grant from Tufts University in the form of a Faculty Summer Research Fellowship, I began the research that eventuated in the basic concept of the book. After initial consultation with Mary Evenson and Mary Barnes, academic fieldwork coordinators in my department, I began interviewing therapists in the greater Boston area. Some of the interviews were done in person and others by telephone. The exact methodology is described in chapter 3. From these interviews, I distilled the complexities of practice. Themes and techniques characteristic of interactive reasoning in occupational therapy result from my analysis. Therapists gave me names of other therapists who became my informants. I was able to discuss the ideas with a group of occupational therapists and individually because of the generosity of James Sellers and his staff at the New England Hospital and Rehabilitation Center in Stoughton, Massachusetts. Pat Keck of the Beth Israel Deaconess Medical Center was generous in identifying several of her staff members as well as herself for interviews. I also discussed my ideas and the project with international colleagues and students during my sabbatical year 1999–2000. My travels took me to Sweden, where with the help of Mona Eklund I was able to discuss interactive reasoning with faculties and students of occupational therapy at the Universities of Lund, Goteborg, and Jonkoping. I also had the opportunity to go to London to discuss these ideas with my colleagues Jennifer A. Butler and Julia Foster-Turner, both faculty members at Oxford Brookes University.

Obviously, this is a skewed sample. The therapists were all interested in the topic, many had studied with my colleagues or me, and all had a personal stake in the topic. It was not a geographically broad sample. The practitioners and faculty were all working in proximity of major academic centers. Nevertheless, what I found was a coherent picture of practice. It is of particular interest to note that this was a particularly tumultuous time for occupational therapists and service delivery agencies in the United States because of cutbacks in Medicare funding. This may reflect the pressured time frame of the practice, but the underlying beliefs remained constant.

Believing in the strong influence of systems on practice, I decided to organize the second portion of the book around practice environments. Although there are other schemes for organizing types of intervention settings, this division flowed naturally from the interviews and underlying conceptual paradigms. In chapter 4, the influence of the medical model is demonstrated in the inpatient and outpatient setting. In chapter 5, The School, one sees a strong influence of an educational model as well as family involvement. In chapter 6, Community, we see a blend of ideas that involve multiple partners in the occupational therapy process. An additional thread central to my thinking is the role of development on interactive issues. This led me to organize the third part of the book around practice populations. Here I clustered age groups into chapters. In chapter 7, the focus is on children and their families; chapter 8, on middle- and later-aged adults, friends, families and partners; and chapter 9, on older adults and caregivers. The young child, older adult, and community move us into what are expected to be growth areas for occupational therapists. Being an educator, I felt it central to conclude the book in part IV with chapter 10 and a look toward the future. The chapter portrays means to education of occupational therapists and research areas for further investigation.

Throughout the book, the reader will see the influence of occupational therapists interviewed for this project. There is no one best way to read this book or make use of the therapist reports. I have organized the information so as to understand three perspectives: (1) the meaning for the person receiving occupational therapy, (2) the recipient's use of the interaction with the therapist, and (3) the therapist's style of presenting therapeutic self to the recipient of care. I welcome the readers to make use of this book in a way that is meaningful to their study and practice.

> Sharan L. Schwartzberg
> 2001
> Boston, Massachusetts

ACKNOWLEDGMENTS

Tufts University, Arts & Sciences, Faculty Research Award, 1999 Summer Research Fellowship

Tufts University Sabbatical Leave 1999–2000

Mark Cohen, Editor

Sarah Brezinsky, Photographer

Nancy Keebler, Writing and Content Consultant

James Foster-Turner, Cover Design

Occupational Therapist (OTR) Practitioner Interviews*

Mary Barnes, University of Massachusetts Medical Center, Worcester, MA; Tufts University, Medford, MA

Sue Brown, St. Joseph's Hospital Southern New England Rehabilitation Center, Warwick, RI

Molly Campbell, Brookline Public Schools, Brookline, MA; Perkins School for the Blind, Watertown, MA

Debbie Caruso, Brookline Public Schools, Brookline, MA

Ellen Cohen Kaplan, Private Practice; Harvard Community Health Plan, Boston, MA

Janet Curran Brooks, Tufts University, Medford, MA

Michael Davison, New England Sinai Hospital and Rehabilitation Center, Stoughton, MA

Regina Doherty, Massachusetts General Hospital, Boston, MA

Kristina Dulberger, Perkins School for the Blind, Watertown, MA

Sherlyn Fenton, St. Camillus Health Center and Hospice, Whittingsville, MA

Merrill Forman, Brookline Public Schools, Brookline, MA

Elizabeth Freeman, Beth Israel Deaconess Medical Center Inpatient Psychiatry, Boston, MA

Kathy Hanlon, Newton Wellesley Hospital Community Education, Newton, MA

Laura Impemba, Health South Braintree Pediatric Rehabilitation at Melrose, MA

Janet Kahane, Newton Wellesley Hospital, Inpatient /Partial Hospital Psychiatry, Newton, MA

Dan Kerls, Newton Wellesley Hospital, Outpatient Rehabilitation Clinic, Newton, MA

Pat Keck, Beth Israel Deaconess Medical Center, Boston, MA

Carol (Harmon) Mahony, Massachusetts General Hospital, Hand Service, Boston, MA

Thayer McCain, Private Practice, Thriving at Home, Medford, MA

Katie McCarthy, Occupational Therapy Associates, Watertown, MA

Linda McGettigan, New England Sinai Hospital and Rehabilitation Center, Stoughton, MA

Michael Nardone, University of Hartford, Hartford, CT

Tom Mercier, Invacare Corporation, New England Region

Mike Miller, Spaulding Rehabilitation Hospital, Boston, MA

Debra Plugis, Framingham Public Schools, Framingham, MA

Kim Quamme, Beth Israel Deaconess Medical Center, Boston, MA

Gary Rabideau, Massachusetts Hospital School, Canton, MA

Sharon Ray, Tufts University, Medford, MA; Private Practice Boston Public Schools, Boston, MA

Rebecca Reynolds, Private Practice; Concord Seabury School, Animals As Intermediaries, Concord, MA

Deborah Rochman, Tufts University, Medford, MA; Tufts Dental School, Gelb Orofacial Pain Center, Boston, MA

Jennifer Saylor, New England Sinai Hospital and Rehabilitation Center, Stoughton, MA

Marion Sitomer, Anne Sullivan Center Early Intervention Program, Lowell, MA

Deborah Slater, New England Baptist Hospital, Boston, MA

Laura Snell, Bay Cove Early Intervention Program, Dorchester, MA

James Sellers, New England Sinai Hospital and Rehabilitation Center, Stoughton, MA

Julie Taberman, New England Sinai Hospital and Rehabilitation Center, Stoughton, MA

Scott A. Trudeau, Edith Nourse Rogers Memorial Veterans Administration Medical Center, Bedford, MA; Tufts University, Medford, MA

Dalit Waller, Neville Manor Nursing Home, Cambridge, MA

Wally VanDyck, St. Joseph's Hospital, Warwick, RI

Case Studies

Mary Barnes

Alice Lowenstein

Mike Miller

Pina Masciarelli-Patel

Sharon Ray

Scott Trudeau

Settings and Therapists Assisting in Photographs

Lisa Brukilacchio, Community Settings, Somerville, MA

Susan Cuervels, Lexington-Arlington-Bedford-Burlington (LABB) School, Lexington High School, Lexington, MA

Regina Doherty, Massachusetts General Hospital, Boston, MA

Faculty and Students Tufts University, Boston School of Occupational Therapy, Medford, MA

Merrill Forman, Brookline Public Schools, Brookline, MA

Rebecca Reynolds, Concord Seabury School, Concord, MA

James Sellers, New England Sinai Hospital and Rehabilitation Center, Stoughton, MA

---

*Employment settings are those at the time interviewed.

Reviewers

Ellen Berger Rainville, Springfield College, Springfield, MA

Liane Hewitt, Loma Linda University, Loma Linda, CA

Patti Kalvelage, Governors State University, University Park, IL

Marianne McArthur, Lake Michigan College, Niles, MI

Judith A. Melvin, Arizona School of Health Sciences, Phoenix, AZ

THE INTERACTIVE REASONING PRACTICE OF OCCUPATIONAL THERAPY

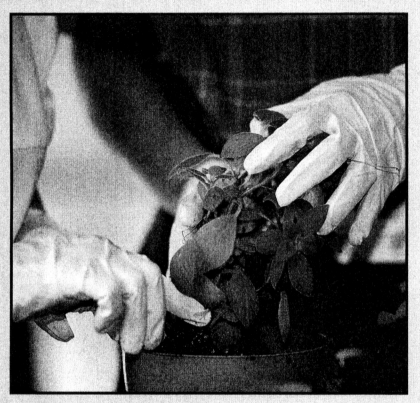

The Power Alliance: An Interactive Reasoning Approach to the Practitioner-Client Relationship

*P*art I **comprises** three chapters that present the foundations of interactive reasoning. Chapter 1 describes the original philosophy of occupational therapy as a phenomenological practice. Chapter 2 follows chronologically with an explanation of ideas borrowed from other fields. Chapter 3 concludes Part I with a detailed description of interactive reasoning as a mode of clinical reasoning as we know it in the modern-day practice of occupational therapy.

THE PHILOSOPHY

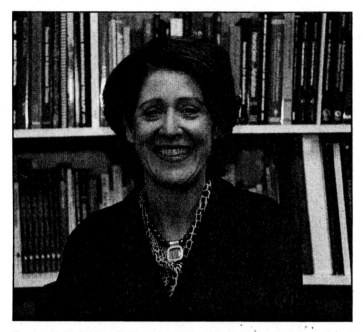

FIGURE 1.1 Values in Humanism: The Philosophy of the Practitioner-Client Relationship

HENRY IN TRANSITION

*H*enry was in a coma for six months after a severe head injury from a car accident. After his rehabilitation program, he was living alone and able to fully care for himself. He is now fifty years old and has been unemployed for several years since the accident. Although he attempted to return to his earlier job as a scientist, his memory problems interfered with his ability to function. He reports being very satisfied with his life and willing to live on a modest income. Most days he spends tending to his finances, taking care of his house, exercising, and maintaining his car. A few weeks ago, he met a woman who has become his regular companion.

OVERVIEW

This chapter describes the philosophy of the interactive domain in occupational therapy, with special emphasis given to ideas from humanistic psychology and phenomenological existential philosophy. These schools of thought are the foundation of the profession's currently favored client-centered approach (Borg & Bruce, 1997). This selection includes theorists repeatedly mentioned or implicitly used by practitioners interviewed for the book. The foundation is drawn from philosophy, psychology, and occupational therapy. As with occupational therapy, a positive relationship exists between ideas of philosophers and the values of psychologists such as Martin Buber and Carl Rogers (Anderson & Cissna, 1997; Friedman, 1965).

The profession's roots are traced back to the philosophical thinking of psychiatrist Adolph Meyer and to nurses, home economists, and others. The client as a whole person—mind, body, and spirit—is considered of importance. From the beginning, occupational therapists valued a life of human occupation balanced through work, play, rest, and sleep as well as quality relationships. The material here does not include everyone who helped form the foundation of how occupational therapists reason and behave in their interactions. The selection is based on therapists' tacit use of the philosophy and high frequency of mention in the occupational therapy literature. Particular emphasis is given to ideas prominent at the time when theory was first being developed in the profession. These beliefs are the foundation of practice as we now know it and act it.

In addition to one-to-one interaction in occupational therapy, group interaction is important. The philosophical tenets and psychological theories underpinning group work in occupational therapy are broad. Interactive reasoning in group work is a specialty area of its own. It is not extensively included here for two reasons. First, therapists primarily focused on one-to-one interactions in the interviews and were not specifically directed to talk about group work in occupational therapy. Second, the reader is directed to other books for full treatment of this subject area (Borg & Bruce, 1991; Cole, 1998; Howe & Schwartzberg, 2001).

THERAPEUTIC RELATIONSHIP THROUGH PROFESSIONAL VALUES IN HUMANISM

THE PHILOSOPHERS

The founding occupational therapists captured the beliefs of several philosophers. Philosophy was central to the original thinking of practitioners as they formulated the foundations of practice. As one can see in the opening case study, human existence is directly influenced by a person's daily functioning, the domain of occupational therapy. Henry's view of the world, the meaningfulness of his sphere of activities, changed directly because of a traumatic and sudden accident.

The philosophers who reflect the profession's points of view include Martin Buber (1965, 1970), Erich Fromm (1992, 1994), and Viktor Frankl (1963, 1986). Buber was foremost in the profession's literature.

Martin Buber: Mutuality and Respect

Martin Buber stands out as the most followed thinker in the writings of occupational therapists, who make repeated references to his ideas. His concepts and meanings gave occupational therapists words to describe the relationship between therapist and client. Buber's view of the "I-Thou" relationship captures the essence of occupational therapists' beliefs in the mutuality between client and therapist.

> Basic words do not state something that might exist outside them; by being spoken they establish a mode of existence.
> Basic words are spoken with one's being.
> When one says You, the I of the word pair I-You is said, too.
> When one says It, the I of the word pair I-It is said, too.
> The basic word I-You can only be spoken with one's whole being.
> The basic word I-It can never be spoken with one's whole being. (Buber, 1970, pp. 53–54)

Buber's (1965) notion of "distance in relation" appears at the base of the client-centered philosophy now practiced. "One should not try to dilute the meaning of the relation: relation is reciprocity" (Buber, 1970, p. 58). The relationship is through "being with" the client by allowing at the same time for connection and separateness. The expectancy of choice and client participation in goal selection exemplifies Buber's philosophy. As Buber stated, "Relation is reciprocity. My You acts on me as I act on it. Our students teach us, our works form us" (1970, p. 67).

One of Buber's (1965) insights is that a principle of human life is twofold, "One movement is the presupposition of the other." Buber explains, "I propose to call the first movement 'the primal setting at a distance' and the second 'entering into relation.' That the first movement is the presupposition of the other is plain from the fact that one can enter into relation only with being which has been set at a distance, more precisely, has become an independent opposite. And it is only for man that an independent opposite exists" (p. 60). In other words, "only when a structure of being is independently over against a living being (Seiende), an independent opposite, does a world exist" (p. 61). Explaining how human life is realized, "distance provides the human situation; relation provides man's becoming in that situation" (p. 64).

Buber also recognized the "normative limits of mutuality" as found in relationships such as those between student and teacher or psychotherapist and client. He describes this partnership as a bipolar situation. As in the case of Henry, as the therapist comes to know him, Henry is at the same time realizing his own potentialities and wishes. (See Critical Case Question 1.1.)

> The teacher who wants to help the pupil to realize his best potentialities must intend him as this particular person, both in his potentiality and in his actuality. More precisely, he must know him not as a mere sum of qualities, aspirations, and inhibitions; he must apprehend him, and affirm him, as a whole. But this he can only do if he encounters him as a partner in a bipolar situation. . . . He must live through this situation in all its aspects not only from his own point of view but

also from that of his partner. He must practice the kind of realization that I call embracing. It is essential that he should awaken the I-You relationship in the pupil, too, who should intend and affirm his educator as this particular person; and yet the educational relationship could not endure if the pupil also practiced the art of embracing by living through the shared situation from the educator's point of view. (Buber, 1970, p. 178)

THERAPEUTIC RELATIONSHIP THROUGH UNDERSTANDING AND ACCEPTANCE

THE PSYCHOLOGISTS

The psychological theory forming central tenets of practice is drawn from original humanistic thinkers such as Frank (1958) on the therapeutic relationship, Carl Rogers (1940/1992, 1957/1992, 1959, 1962, 1965) on client-centered therapy, Abraham Maslow (1954/1987, 1968) on the hierarchy of needs and self-actualization, Erik Erikson (1984) on psychosocial stages of development, Robert White (1959, 1971) on the "urge toward competence" and, more recently, Csikszentmihalyi (1975, 1990, 1993, 1996; Csikszentmihalyi & Csikszentmihalyi, 1988) on the "flow state." Psychodynamic theory must also be included for contributions to understanding of the unconscious and counter-transference (Freud, 1949, 1960a, 1960b). Occupational therapists also broadly apply object-relations theory for ideas on development (Mahler, 1968; Mahler, Pine, & Bergman, 1975; Winnicott, 1965, 1971, 1987, 1988) and interpersonal-relations theory for ways of understanding communication (Sullivan, 1953, 1954) as well as personality dynamics (Horney, 1937, 1939, 1945, 1950). Chapter 2, The Borrowed Practice, includes current theorists who directly concern themselves with the therapeutic relationship, as do other chapters where relevant, for example, family systems theory.

Again, when they speak about their reasoning in the interactive domain, occupational therapists often draw upon psychological principles. Regrettably, they do not frequently give attribution by naming the original theorists or by using the original language and terminology. However, they do apply the theory in their thinking and actions. In the following summary, the theorists are for the most part presented in the order of their prominence as reference points in occupational therapy.

Jerome Frank: Therapeutic Use and Awareness of Self

Over forty years ago Frank (1958), a psychiatrist, was invited to speak to occupational therapists on the therapeutic use of self. He approached this task by exploring two related topics: (1) the relationship between the perceptual and behavioral aspects of the client's self and (2) the therapist's use of self as a therapeutic tool. His point of view appears grounded in an existential and humanistic philosophy.

Frank observed the power of expectancies in influencing bodily states, thinking, feeling, as well as action. He stated, "From the fact that each of us constructs a world based on his expectancies, it follows that to the extent that we can influence another person's expectancies, we can affect how he feels, thinks and behaves" (p. 216). Frank identified three selves that are developed from interactions with others and the resultant successes and failures: (1) the acting self, (2) the perceived self, and (3) the ideal self. He points out that a person cannot directly perceive his or her own acting self, but rather, the person perceives the responses of others to the roles the person plays.

Frank explains that although the nature and extent of a person's disability are important in determining a person's self-image, it is the way the person perceives the disability that is more important. In the chapter-opening case, Henry perceives his new life as satisfying. This requires him to shed old images of others' definitions of success and his own picture of his ideal self.

In referring to the *transference reaction*, Frank notes, "Our patients cannot see themselves as others see them, because they see themselves as others *saw* them, and they are unable to shake themselves loose from this image" (p. 219). He explains that the three ways, in spite of experiences otherwise, we maintain the constancy of this picture of our self-image are (1) avoidance, (2) selective inattention, and (3) self-fulfilling prophecy (p. 219). In situations where parents reflect a derogatory or inconsistent picture to the child, the result is a self-image that is disorganized and not readily changed because of residual anxiety. Clients commonly present three profiles or self-disturbances: (1) difficulties in the acting self, (2) difficulties with the perceived self, and (3) discrepancies between the perceived, acting, and ideal selves (p. 220). According to Frank, it is the discrepancies between the selves that plague people, for example, the tendency to underestimate one's acting self—the discrepancy between the ideal self and the perceived self.

For the therapist, the task, according to Frank, is to present an acting self to the client that allows him or her to achieve a better integration of self. Frank cautions that the therapist keep the therapeutic role distinct or risk therapeutic efficiency. For example, one risk is trying too hard to help because of high expectations. This can arouse false expectations and feed into excessive dependency. If not successful, the therapist puts him or herself at risk of becoming frustrated and reacting with anger. Frank states, "The therapeutic role of the occupational therapist is confined to trying to bring about modifications in the acting self of the patient" (p. 223). The occupational therapist's task is to help strengthen the client's healthy aspects by acting in a way to "disappoint his pathological expectancies" (p. 223). This calls for what Frank terms *predictable flexibility*, being consistent in what is the most consistent role, leaving room for flexibility and spontaneity (p. 224). In the therapeutic use of self, "it must be different enough to arouse an optimal amount of anxiety in the patient, since this is a powerful stimulus to learning, but not so different as to arouse excessive anxiety, which is paralyzing and serves merely to reinforce the patient's original behavior" (p. 224). Frank concludes by saying, "One of the tasks of the occupational therapist is to use himself to help the patient develop a more workable self of his own. . . . To use himself effectively the therapist must also have a clear realization of his own abilities and limitations" (p. 224).

Carl Rogers: Therapeutic Conditions of Genuineness, Empathy, and Positive Regard

Central to occupational therapists' philosophy are beliefs based upon the work of Carl Rogers. His view of the conditions central to the personality change and his definitions of *empathy* as well as *therapist's genuineness* (1957/1992) are ideas common to the culture of occupational therapy. (See Information Checkpoint 1.1

and Key Terms.) The value placed on empathy has weathered shifts in theoretical and service orientations of the profession. Nevertheless, empathy, as Rogers (1952/1957) explained it, remains key to the profession's thinking about the therapeutic process: "To sense the client's private world as if it were your own, but without ever losing the 'as if' quality—this is empathy, and this seems essential to therapy" (p. 829). (See Critical Case Question 1.2.)

Abraham Maslow: Human Impulse toward Self-Actualization and Wellness

Maslow's work is widely applied to understand human motivation. Occupational therapists have liberally drawn from his work originally published in 1954, again in 1970, and finally in 1987. Maslow was a major force in humanistic psychology. Believing that individuals have the tendency to move to higher levels of health and fulfillment, he supported a holistic view of people and their ability to self-actualize (Maslow, 1987). His ideas remain to this day central to the profession's thinking. The principles often drawn upon include the following:

- "Let us emphasize that it is unusual, *not* usual, for an act or a conscious wish to have but one motivation" (p. 6). "The clinical psychologists have long since found that any behavior may be a channel through which flow various impulses. Or to say it in another way, most behavior is overdetermined or multimotivated. Within the sphere of motivational determinants any behavior tends to be determined by several or *all* of the basic needs simultaneously rather than by only one of them. The latter would be more an exception than the former" (p. 29).
- Basic needs are arranged in a hierarchy of less or greater priority or potency. "Relative gratification submerges them and allows the next higher set of needs in the hierarchy to emerge, dominate, and organize the personality. . ." (p. 32). "*At once other (and higher) needs emerge* and these, rather than physiological hungers, dominate the organism. And when these in turn are satisfied, again new (and still higher) needs emerge, and so on. This is what we mean by saying that the basic human needs are organized into a hierarchy of relative prepotency" (p. 17).
- "But a want that is satisfied is no longer a want. The organism is dominated and its behavior organized only by unsatisfied needs. . . . This statement is somewhat qualified by a hypothesis . . . that it is precisely those individuals in whom a certain need has always been satisfied who are best equipped to tolerate deprivation of that need in the future and that, furthermore, those who have been deprived in the past will react differently to current satisfactions from the one who has never been deprived" (p. 18).
- The basic needs hierarchy, in order, includes physiological needs, safety needs, belongingness and love needs, esteem needs, and self-actualization need. Some other needs Maslow identified, although rarely made explicit but imbued in the occupational therapist's thinking, include the cognitive need or impulse, desire to know and to understand, and aesthetic needs.

Erik Erikson: Life Stage Crises from Infancy to Old Age

The profession's foundation for understanding human development is derived from Erikson's epigenetic scheme of psychosocial development (Erikson, 1984). The concept of *life cycle*, or epigenesis, forces therapists to think of the whole course of life. This course relates the last stage to the first stage in relation to the course of individuals and to that of generations. We are most likely unaware that our views are based in Erikson's idea that life stages are dominated by both a syntonic and a dystonic quality. At each stage, there are essential developments. Together they constitute a "crisis" in that the "syntonic should systematically outweigh or at least balance (but never dismiss) the dystonic" (p. 157). Erikson further explains that "the final balance of all stages of development must leave the syntonic elements dominant in order to secure a *basic strength* emerging from each overall crisis: at the beginning, it is Hope, and, at the end, what we are calling Wisdom" (p. 159). As occupational therapists view the interaction of developmental needs of individuals, they are likely using Erikson's stages as a point of reference. (See Information Checkpoint 1.2.) (See Critical Case Question 1.3.)

Robert White: Effectance and the Human Urge towards Competence

In 1971, Robert White wrote his much applied and quoted paper "The Urge towards Competence" published in the *American Journal of Occupational Therapy*. Over thirty years ago, he was concerned with shortened treatment and a growing focus on efficiency. Foreseeing issues that are even more acute today, White warned occupational therapists to be alert to the client's sense of competence. He saw competence as pivotal to self-esteem and dependent upon a sense of confidence that one can make things happen. The effect is that others appreciate and recognize competence. The recognition then feeds into a person's sense of self-esteem. White observed that "the encouragement of performances that will increase efficacy and confidence is a formula that applies generally to many aspects of helping" (p. 274). Later in this book, we will see occupational therapists echo these sentiments as they describe their interactive reasoning.

Mihaly Csikszentmihalyi: Just Right Challenge and Flow State

A flow state occurs when the demands of the situation present a "just right," or optimal, challenge leading to satisfaction (Csikszentmihalyi, 1975). The positive match or mismatch between skills and challenge occurs in everyday activities. Extrapolating to the therapeutic relationship, occupational therapists are interested in providing the optimal match between the client, the activity, and the interaction.

Csikszentmihalyi (1990) believes that people experience a flow state when their "skills match with the opportunities for action in the environment" (p. 177). He calls this an "optimal experience" (p. 3)—"a sense that one's skills are adequate to cope with the challenges at hand, in a goal-directed, rule-bound, action system that provides clear clues as to how well one is performing. Concentration is so intense that there is no attention left to think about anything irrelevant, or to worry about problems" (p. 71).

Sigmund Freud: Mental Life and Individual Development

Freud took the position that mental life, or our psyche, is made up of several parts. Through studying individual development he identified the parts or what he called psychical agencies: the id, the ego, and the superego (1949, pp. 14–15). The ego has the task of preservation by taking over the demands of the instincts; the id, by either allowing satisfaction, postponing satisfaction, or "suppressing their excitations entirely" (p. 15). "The raising of tensions is in general felt as *unpleasure* and their lowering as *pleasure*. . . . An increase in unpleasure that is expected and foreseen is met by a *signal of anxiety*; the occasion of such an increase, whether it threatens from without or within, is known as *danger*" (p. 15). Following the child's prolonged period of dependence on the parent, as Freud explains, the parental influence remains as a remnant called the superego (p. 15). The function of the ego is to simultaneously satisfy the demands of reality, the id, and the superego. Otherwise put, "the ego represents what may be called reason and common sense, in contrast to the id, which contains the passions" (Freud, 1960a, p. 15).

Freud, through his studies of the child's attachment to mother, gives us the concept of *identification*. Although now widely protested, the idea stems from his idea of the little girl's first wish, or "penis envy." The girl abandons her loved mother because she cannot forgive her for not having a penis. "In her resentment over this she gives up her mother and puts someone else in her place as the object of her love—her father. If one has lost a love-object, the most obvious reaction is to identify oneself with it, to replace it from within, as it were, by identification. . . . Identification with her mother can take the place of attachment to her mother" (1960a, pp. 76–77).

Reality testing is a term often heard in occupational therapy. It can be traced to Freud's discussion of the "reality principle." Freud stated, "Just as the id is directed exclusively to obtaining pleasure, so the ego is governed by considerations of safety. The ego has set itself the task of self-preservation, which the id appears to neglect" (1949, p. 86). Freud goes on to explain that there is the possibility of confusion which gives way to mistaking of reality. The ego, he further explains guards against this possibility through reality testing. Freud stated, "Since memory-traces can become conscious just as perceptions do, especially through their association with residues of speech, the possibility arises of a confusion which would lead to a mistaking of reality" (p. 86). Because of the special conditions of sleep, the ego lets go of reality testing in dreams, he explains.

To understand Freud's (1960a) notion of the unconscious one must understand repression. Freud stated, "The state in which the ideas existed before being made conscious is called by us *repression*, and we assert that the force which instituted the repression and maintains it is perceived as *resistance* during the work of analysis" (p. 4). He went on to explain, "The repressed is the prototype of the unconscious for us. We see, however, that we have two kinds of unconscious—the one which is latent but capable of becoming conscious, and the one which is repressed and which is not, in itself and without more ado, capable of becoming conscious. . . . The latent, which is unconscious only descriptively, not in the dynamic sense, we call *preconscious*. . . ." (p. 5).

The idea that something like forgetting a proper name is not just forgetting but has other meanings can well be attributed to Freud (1960b). Such forgetting, he explains, has a *motive* in the process. To forget a proper name is perhaps to want to forget something else that is wanted to be forgotten and is repressed. Freud also elaborated on other acts such as slips of the tongue, errors, and bungled actions that he explained at the level of the unconscious. These explanations have become common to the American culture of understanding. The interpretation of unconscious motives now often serves as a source of joking and emotional release in ordinary conversation. Memory loss, a possible neurological sequel of brain damage, such as in the case of Henry, should be distinguished from the psychological state of repression.

Karen Horney: Culture and Conflict

Horney (1937) stated, "The conception of what is normal varies not only with the culture but also within the same culture, in the course of time" (p.15). She criticized Freud for being rooted in his scientific orientations and suggested we take a step beyond his overemphasis on the biological origin of mental characteristics; that is, instinctual drives and object relationships are biologically determined by human nature or arise out of unalterable situations like the biologically given pregenital stages, Oedipus complex. She explained that life conditions in every culture give rise to some fears and that the fears existing in a culture are warded off in ways such as taboos, customs, and rites. For example, "the direct outcome of the anxiety involved in neurotic competitiveness is a fear of failure and a fear of success" (p. 211). Further, "from its economic center competition radiates into all other activities and permeates love, social relations and play. Therefore competition is a problem for everyone in our culture, and it is not at all surprising to find it an unfailing center of neurotic conflicts" (p. 188). Horney (1939), in a radical effort at the time, demonstrated how Freud erred.

Horney (1945) stated that externalization is the "tendency to experience internal processes as if they occurred outside oneself and, as a rule, to hold these external factors as responsible for one's difficulties. It has in common with idealization the purpose of getting away from the real self" (p. 115). With neurotic symptoms are underlying conflicts. Horney identifies tendencies or types of ways people deal with basic conflict or faces of conflict: compliant type: "moving toward people," the aggressive type: "moving against people," and the detached type: "moving away from people." One way the neurotic attempts to solve conflicts is by repressing certain aspects of the personality and bringing the opposite out into the fore, and another is by putting distance between him or herself and others. The idealized image and externalization are attempts to get away from the real self. There then exists a protective structure that is rigid. The person fears that "equilibrium will be disturbed" and also has a "fear of exposure." There is the "waste of human energies" in the form of "ineffectualness," "the pretense of love," "the pretense of goodness, unselfishness, sympathy" (p. 164), "the pretense of interest and knowledge," "the pretense of honesty and fairness" (especially in aggressive types with marked sadistic trends), "the pretense of suffering" (p. 165), "unconscious arrogance" (p. 167), "the inability to take a definite stand" and the "undependability that goes along with it" (p. 168). "Hopelessness is an ultimate product of unresolved conflicts, with its deepest root in the despair of ever being wholehearted and undivided" (p. 183).

In summary, Horney (1940) explains ways that neurotics relieve tension. Compulsive forces are driving these individuals, resulting "in active moves away from the real self and against it" (p. 177).

Harry Stack Sullivan: Structure and Process in the Interview

Our understanding of the concept of anxiety as the main disruptive element in interpersonal relations can be attributed to Sullivan (1953). Sullivan's theory was that "the tension of anxiety, when present in the mothering one, induces anxiety in the infant" (p. 41). Sullivan explained that both early in life and later in life there are two types of tensions: tensions of needs and tensions of anxiety. The former can be satisfied and can be experienced as fear of the danger of the need, and the latter is elicited by an "interpersonal situation," hence the need for interpersonal security.

As the self develops, it becomes organized in a way to protect against feelings of anxiety. Sullivan says, "The self-system thus is an organization of educative experience called into being by the necessity to avoid or to minimize incidents of anxiety" (p. 165). He further explains that in maladaptive situations children may be treated hurtfully when they need tenderness, when they do things that may have once brought caring. This denial of caring provokes anxiety. The child eventually perceives the need for tenderness as anxiety or pain. Rather than show the need to authority figures, the child shows a negative attitude. "The other elaborations—the malevolence that shows as a basic attitude toward life, you might say, as a profound problem in one's interpersonal relations—are also just an elaboration of this earlier warp" (pp. 214–215). The choice of intervention is for the patient to be able to identify the situation that provoked anxiety. From this observation, inference is made about the pattern of corresponding interpersonal difficulty. Sullivan recognizes that this is a difficult task but not impossible. The challenge becomes greater when the patient's personality system has an actual disassociation. The person will then have tremendous difficulty remembering significant aspects of the actual situation that evoked the anxiety.

Sullivan (1954) offered therapists a structure and process for interpersonal exchange called the "psychiatric interview." He (1953) listened to his patients in an attempt to understand: How does the threat of anxiety affect the patient's interpersonal communication and daily life situations? Since his original work, many have written about interviewing. Sullivan was clear in communicating the technical aspects of an interview. For example, he said, "To sum up, the smooth transition is used to move gently to a new topic; the accented transition saves time and clarifies the situation; and the abrupt transition is ordinarily used either to avoid dangerous anxiety or to provoke anxiety where you can't get anywhere otherwise" (1954, p. 49). In addition to offering a method to transitions in an interview, he gave a developmental framework to the phases of an interview, for example, early stages, detailed inquiry, and termination of the interview. The topics he suggested in his outline for obtaining data should be very familiar to the modern-day occupational therapist. Sullivan included topics such as, in his words, disorders in learning toilet habits, attitudes toward games and partners in them, attitudes toward competition and compromise, ambition, initial schooling, attitude toward solitude, eating habits, sleep and sleep functions, the sex life, vocational history, and avocational interests. Many of his topics make up the modern-day occupational therapy history or occupational history.

Donald W. Winnicott: Nature of Attachment and Transitional Objects

A pediatrician and adult and child analyst, Winnicott is most often quoted for his work in describing the psychological development of the infant (1965) and the role of instinct in human development (1988). He coined several terms and concepts that are in common use among therapists, educators, and others interested in human development. Those reviewed here include *good-enough mother* (1965), *transitional object* (1965), the *depressive position* (1988), and *holding* (1972).

Winnicott (1965) portrayed early infant attachment as a "relationship to part-objects" (p. 10). For example, the baby relates to a breast, the mother not being a full person but "known" at contacts that are affectionate. Winnicott categorizes the good-enough mother (p. 18) as having three functions in the early stage of the child's life by creating a "facilitating environment" (p. 19). These functions include

(1) holding, (2) handling, and (3) object presenting (realizing, making real the infant's creative impulse, capability to relate to objects (p. 18). Winnicott concludes, "My thesis is that what we do in therapy is to attempt to imitate the natural process that characterizes the behaviour of any mother of her own infant. If I am right, it is the mother-infant couple that can teach us the basic principles on which we may base our therapeutic work, when we are treating children whose early mothering was 'not good enough', or was interrupted" (pp. 19–20).

Winnicott (1965) firmly believed that by understanding the normal child's enjoyment we could understand the needs of the deprived child. He explains that if a child is deprived of transitional objects, the only way out for the child is to develop a split in the personality. One-half of the personality is related to the child's subjective world, and the other to the world that is impinging and to which the child must comply.

Winnicott (1965) also explains that children who are maladapted either have not had a transitional object or have lost it. He further explains that "there must be someone for the object to stand for, which means that the condition of these children cannot be cured simply by giving them a new object" (p. 144). The child develops a "false self" so as to make contact with the environment and hide the "true self" (p. 153).

Winnicott (1971) makes a clear stance and contribution with his view that play is essential to psychotherapy. He explains that the therapist must be able to play to be suited to the work. For the work of therapy to occur, the patient needs to be able to play. It is from the vantage point of play that the creativity needed for therapy to evolve will ensue. Winnicott empathetically states that "psychotherapy has to do with two people playing together" (p. 38).

Margaret S. Mahler: Therapy As a Corrective Developmental Experience

Through her observations of the pre-school-age child with psychosis, Mahler (1968) came to explain early human development and corollary principles of treatment. She proposed that the therapist's role is to substitute for ego function in the child. In addition, when the child is ready, the therapist's function is to educate about social relationships. In sum, the therapist provides a corrective mothering experience. We will later see that these concepts are basic to the thinking of occupational therapists.

More specifically, Mahler believed that in development it is normal for the child to go through an autistic and symbiotic phase as well as a separation-individuation phase. Mahler said, "We postulate that in the normal autistic phase, the infant is not yet aware of anything beyond his own body, whereas in the symbiotic phase he seems to have become vaguely aware that need satisfaction comes from the outside. The mother is still, however, a part of his own self-representation: the infant's mental image is fused with that of his mother. In the third phase (the period of separation-individuation), the infant gradually becomes aware of his separateness: first, the separateness of his body, then gradually the entity and identity of his self, as he establishes its core and boundaries" (p. 165). (See Information Checkpoint 1.3.)

Mahler postulated that in treatment of the psychotic child the therapist become the "auxiliary ego" in substitution for missed or unsatisfactory development (p. 170). She believed this process would enable the child to restore ego functions, establish an integrated body image, and develop object relationships. Mahler's theory aimed to have the child reexperience missed stages of development: presymbiotic, symbiotic, and separation-individuation.

In summary, the therapist's role, according to Mahler, is to (1) facilitate the living and working through of early developmental phases, providing the lacking ego functions necessary to the development of self-concept, (2) protect the child against excessive stimulation, (3) engage the child in a common purpose to divert the child's attention away from threatening inner stimuli, and (4) delve into the primary process type of symbolic behavior without anxiety and with empathy that allows for reality testing in differentiating between inner and outer environments. (See Information Checkpoint 1.4.) The prior is done with "firm definition of limits and boundaries in both the play situation and the interpersonal relationship" (p. 175).

THERAPEUTIC RELATIONSHIP THROUGH AUTHENTIC AND MEANINGFUL OCCUPATION

THE OCCUPATIONAL THERAPISTS

The earlier works of three occupational therapists seriously considered the nature of the therapeutic relationship in occupational therapy and built upon the thinking of the psychologists and philosophers. Gail Fidler spoke on a "communication process in psychiatry" (Fidler & Fidler, 1963) and coined "doing and becoming: purposeful action and self-actualization" (Fidler & Fidler, 1978). Elizabeth Yerxa (1967) brought to the field the concept of authentic occupational therapy. Ann Mosey's contribution is significant for her developmental group theory (1970) emanating from recapitulation of ontogenesis (1968), therapeutic use of activities (1973), and her outline of the "legitimate tools" in her "configuration of a profession" occupational therapy (1981). Howe and Schwartzberg's (1995; 2001) work is highlighted as a theoretical foundation for group work in occupational therapy. Finally, Gary Kielhofner's (1983, 1985, 1995) work on the model of human occupation, fondly called "MOHO," is essential to understanding both novice and experienced therapists' views on human occupation originally drawn from Mary Reilly's (1966, 1969) concept of occupational behavior. This section places a heavy emphasis on occupational therapists viewed historically as primarily contributing to the psychosocial area of practice. More recent work on client-centered and family-centered practice is addressed in later discussions of the therapeutic relationship in occupational therapy.

Gail Fidler: Doing and Becoming through Purposeful Action

In developing her work, Fidler refers to Erikson's (Fidler & Fidler, 1978) valuing "doing" in a person's developing a sense of mastery, personal integrity, and success in the external world. In this same paper, she also grounds her ideas in White's thesis of the innate human drive to master the environment as motivation toward competence. Fidler concludes, "There is an accumulation of significant data to support the thesis that the drive to action, transformed into the ability to 'do,' is fundamental to ego development and adaptation" (p. 306).

Elizabeth Yerxa: Authentic Occupational Therapy

One can firmly surmise that what Yerxa (1967) defined as *authentic occupational therapy* is well accepted as a definition. Yerxa identified four essential aspects of occupational therapy that identify the profession's uniqueness. (See Information Checkpoint 1.5.) "Occupational therapy is unique because we use the choice of self-initiated purposeful activities to produce a reality-orienting influence upon the client's perception of himself and his environment so he can function" (p. 3). Yerxa further explained that our view of people agrees with some of the existential thinkers, namely Martin Buber. "Personal authenticity as an occupational therapist means that the therapist allows himself to feel real emotion as he enters into *mutual* relation with the client. . . . The authentic occupational therapist is involved in the process of caring and to care means to be affected just as surely as it means to affect" (p. 8).

Ann Mosey: Conscious Use of Self and Activities

Mosey (1981) identifies what she calls six "legitimate tools of occupational therapy": the nonhuman environment, conscious use of self, teaching-learning process, purposeful activities, activity groups, and activity analysis and synthesis. Mosey (1986) explains that "conscious use of self includes but is greater than rapport and the art of practice" (p. 199). She points out that this is a conscious manipulation of responses to help the client in a group, in a one-to-one relationship, or with significant others. Mosey draws upon Martin Buber to explain the complexity of the relationship between therapist and client. She identifies several therapist qualities that enable the use of self as a tool. (See Information Checkpoint 1.6.)

Mosey (1970) carefully explains the developmental nature of the therapeutic process in occupational therapy. Her developmental theory is based on three postulates: (1) "deviations in development can be altered," (2) "subskills fundamental to mature adaptive skills must be acquired in a sequential manner," and (3) "mature adaptive skills can be acquired through participation in situations that simulate those interactions believed to be responsible for the sequential development of a given adaptive skill" (p. 272). Mosey identifies five types of developmental groups: parallel, project, egocentric cooperative, cooperative, and mature (p. 272). The developmental groups are structured to lead to adaptive skills in group interaction. Some of the therapist methods used to encourage desired behavior at the various levels include reinforcing approximated behaviors, modeling and encouraging imitation, suggestion and encouragement from group members and the leader, and experimentation. Mosey suggests that as a heuristic device, the concept of developmental groups can also be useful in treatment of other adaptive skills. This schema remains to this day broadly applied in occupational therapy practice.

Howe and Schwartzberg: Adaptation through Action in the Functional Group

The functional approach to group work is described by Howe and Schwartzberg (1995, 2001) as a generic model for occupational therapists. The therapist, in this case, group leader, employs techniques to encourage adaptive action that is purposeful, self-initiated, spontaneous, or here and now, and group centered. The therapeutic use of self includes leader skills such as planning the group activity, genuineness, empathy, modeling behavior, reality testing, and communication. In communicating, the therapist follows strategies of listening and responding, giving and receiving feedback, concreteness, and confrontation. Observation of functioning of the individuals, such as roles assumed in the group, the group as a whole, and the former in relation to the activity, is key to making judgements about the therapist's use of self.

Mary Reilly: Occupation As Therapeutic Milieu

In 1966, Reilly recognized the "unique patient-occupational therapy relationship" that occurs in "clear cut work-play settings." She stated, "It operates from the specialized knowledge which an occupational therapist has about psychiatric communication. It has in the relationship certain additional characteristics concerned with the transactions which go on between the patient, the therapist and his creative product and between the patient, his therapist and the psychological contract a patient makes with tasks and job" (pp. 66–67). In her vision of the therapeutic milieu, Reilly also drew upon Maslow's hierarchical classification of basic human needs. She believed the milieu should acknowledge competency, arouse curiosity, and satisfy human need states through occupation. The theoretical framework guiding her model (Reilly, 1969) also drew upon the contributions of psychologists such as Robert White, Eric Erikson, and David McClelland. The frame supported the belief in achievement, its developmental underpinnings, and the concept of role, learned in the process of socialization, as the theoretical basis of occupational therapy.

Role changes are addressed in occupational therapy. The meaning of activities may change for a person who becomes ill or disabled. In the case of Henry, aspects of his self-care have become his work. Therapist sensitivity to necessary changes in patterns of occupational behavior is central to establishing an empathic relationship.

Gary Kielhofner: Occupation as Human Motivational and Organizational Force

The model of human occupation (MOHO) (Kielhofner, 1997; Kielhofner & Nicol, 1989) as articulated by Kielhofner and his associates "addresses the motivation for occupation, the patterning of occupational behavior into routines and lifestyles, the nature of skilled performance, and the influence of environment on occupational behavior" (Kielhofner, 1997, p. 187). Occupational therapists draw upon this frame to look at the person in context of his or her whole life, that is, roles, habits, daily patterns, and interests. (See Information Checkpoint 1.7.) The information serves to give definition to what questions to raise and to understanding the client's values, daily life, and expectations. (See Critical Case Question 1.4.)

Therapists routinely apply the model as a guide to explain a client's circumstances and as a framework for program development. Because the concepts are so widely applied, the model has become central to the occupational therapist's ways of thinking in formulating the direction of interactions and evaluations. The concepts are reflected in the types of data collected, both through structured protocols and interviews and as the focus of informal interactions (Kielhofner, 1997).

BACK TO HENRY

One can view Henry's story from a variety of perspectives. Philosophy tells the occupational therapist to understand Henry through his view of the world. Psychology offers an explanation about ways to understand Henry's motivation and drives. Through an examination of Henry's early life experiences and attachments, his relationships to people, work, and nonhuman objects will be better understood. Finally, occupational therapy principles help to explain Henry in the occupational context of his changed world of new activities, challenges, and roles.

SUMMARY

Philosophers, psychologists, and occupational therapists laid down the foundations of interactive reasoning. Central themes were derived from humanistic values. These tenets, respecting the individual and belief in the growth potential of all people, inform the manner of style in occupational therapy interactions that are client centered.

REFLECTIVE QUESTIONS

- Describe the philosophical thinking that drives occupational therapy interactions. How does the philosophy influence practice? Reflect upon your own philosophical beliefs. How are they congruent with those maintained in occupational therapy, or are they significantly different?
- Several psychological theories guide occupational therapy practice. In what ways do these theories explain the ways occupational therapists interact with clients and students? As you think about these concepts, identify their relevance to your own life and potential areas for growth as well as self-understanding.
- Several occupational therapists help form the ways of relating in the profession. Who were these therapists, and what was their unique contribution? In reflecting upon their contribution to our understanding of the therapeutic relationship, are there other occupational therapy theorists you would add to those reviewed, and what points of view do they represent?

INFORMATION CHECKPOINTS

1.1. NECESSARY AND SUFFICIENT CONDITIONS OF THERAPEUTIC PERSONALITY CHANGE

"For constructive personality change to occur, it is necessary that these conditions exist and continue over a period of time:

- Two persons are in psychological contact.
- The first, whom we shall term the client, is in a state of incongruence, being vulnerable or anxious.

- The second person, whom we shall term the therapist, is congruent or integrated in the relationship.
- The therapist experiences unconditional positive regard for the client.
- The therapist experiences an empathic understanding of the client's internal frame of reference and endeavors to communicate this experience to the client.
- The communication to the client of the therapist's empathic understanding and unconditional positive regard is to a minimal degree achieved" (C. R. Rogers, 1957/1992, p. 827).

1.2. STAGES OF PSYCHOSOCIAL DEVELOPMENT (ERIKSON, 1984)

Infancy	Basic trust versus basic mistrust (hope)
Early childhood	Autonomy versus shame, doubt (will)
Play age	Initiative versus guilt (purpose)
School age	Industry versus inferiority (competence)
Adolescence	Indentity versus confusion (fidelity)
Young adulthood	Intimacy versus isolation (love)
Adulthood	Generativity versus stagnation (care)
Old age	Integrity versus despair (wisdom)

1.3. DEVELOPMENT OF A SENSE OF IDENTITY

"Normal separation-individuation is the first crucial prerequisite for the development and maintenance of the 'sense of identity'" (Mahler, Pine, & Bergman, 1975, p. 11).

1.4. SCHEME OF THE PHASES OF SEPARATION-INDIVIDUATION PROCESS (MAHLER, PINE, & BERGMAN, 1975)

- Forerunners: Normal autistic and symbiotic holding phase.
- First subphase: Differentiation and the development of body image ("hatching," transitional objects, "the checking back pattern," and "stranger anxiety") (four to eight months).
- Second subphase: Practicing (crawling to upright locomotion, "peek-a-boo") (ten or twelve months to sixteen or eighteen months).
- Third subphase: Rapprochement (renewed need for closeness—"shadowing and darting-away practices" (fifteen to twenty-four months).
- Fourth subphase: Consolidation of individuality and the beginnings of emotional object constancy (twenty-five to twenty-eight months).

1.5. FOUR ASPECTS OF OCCUPATIONAL THERAPY'S UNIQUENESS (YERXA, 1967, P. 3)

1. Choice
2. Self-initiated purposeful activity
3. Reality orientation of client's potential
4. Reality-orienting influence on perception of physical environment, psychological self, social self

1.6. THERAPIST QUALITIES THAT ENABLE CONSCIOUS USE OF SELF (MOSEY, 1986, PP. 200–202)

- Perception of individuality
- Respect for the dignity and rights of each individual
- Empathy
- Compassion

- Humility
- Unconditional positive regard
- Honesty
- A relaxed manner
- Flexibility
- Self-awareness
- Humor
- Collaborative ability

1.7. Model of Occupational Behavior

"Engaging in occupational behavior:

- Maintains, restores, reorganizes, or develops capacities, motives, and life styles
- Transforms people into more adaptive and healthy beings" (Kielhofner, 1997, p. 212).

Critical Case Questions

1.1. Henry is not working. What concerns would you, as an occupational therapist, have about his existence? Would you directly express them to Henry or take a different approach in the first meeting?

1.2. If you imagined Henry's world "as if it were your own," how would you describe Henry's daily existence?

1.3. Consider Henry's developmental stage in life and his potential for self-actualization. Describe how you would imagine his life as he leads it to its fullest potential.

1.4. If you were to meet Henry, what curiosity would you, as an occupational therapist, have about his life, for example, habits, roles, associations?

Key Terms

Developmental Group Levels (Mosey, 1970)

- Parallel group: "An aggregate of patients who are involved in individual tasks with the minimal necessity for interaction. . . . The therapist provides assistance with tasks and takes responsibility for meeting the social-emotional needs of each member" (pp. 272–273).
- Project group: "Members are involved in common, short-term tasks that require some interaction, cooperation, and competition. The task is paramount. Mutual interaction outside the task is not expected. The therapist provides, or assists the group in selecting, tasks that require interaction of two or more persons for completion. He responds to the social-emotional needs of group members" (p. 273).
- Egocentric-cooperative group: "Characterized by group members selecting, implementing, and executing relatively long-term tasks through joint

interaction. The task remains central but satisfaction of some social-emotional needs of fellow group members is encouraged. . . . The therapist gives support and guidance relative to the task and continues to satisfy a considerable portion of each member's social-emotional needs" (p. 273).

- Cooperative group: "Members are encouraged to identify and gratify each other's social-emotional needs in conjunction with task accomplishment. This type of group often includes only members of the same sex. The therapist acts primarily in the role of advisor and may not be present at all group meetings" (p. 273).
- Mature group: "Heterogeneous in composition and characterized by members taking those task and social-emotional roles that are required for adequate group functioning. Maintenance of a proper balance between productivity and personal need satisfaction is stressed. The therapist acts as a coequal member" (p. 273).

Authentic Occupational Therapy

"Authentic occupational therapy is based upon a *commitment* to the client's realization of his own particular meaning. The authentic occupational therapist recognizes that although initial dependency might require a temporary suspension of the patient's right to choice, the therapeutic experience is primarily an opportunity for self-actualization. Therefore, the occupational therapist does not force his value system upon the client. But rather, through using his skills and knowledge, [he] exposes the client to a range of possibilities which constitute his external reality. The client is the one who makes the choice" (Yerxa, 1967, p. 8).

Competence

The natural tendency toward dealing with the environment is fundamental to human behavior, explains Robert White. "To be competent means to be sufficient or adequate to meet the demands of a situation or task. . . . The evolutionary importance of such an urge is not difficult to discern" (White, 1971, p. 273).

Conscious Use of Self

"Conscious use of self involves a planned interaction with another person in order to alleviate fear or anxiety; provide reassurance; obtain necessary information; provide information; give advice; and assist the other individual to gain more appreciation, expression, and functional use of his or her latent inner resources. Such a relationship is concerned with promoting growth and development, improving and maintaining function, and fostering a greater ability to cope with the stresses of life" (Mosey, 1981, pp. 95–96).

The Depressive Position in Emotional Development

This is a state in normal development where there is integration of quiet and excited, the infant's guilt feelings or concern about relationships because of the instinctual (excited) elements. It is not referring to a clinically depressed mood. Rather, it refers to a stage of development in the healthy infant's ability to mourn loss. "The important thing is the infant's or the individual's new capacity to accept responsibility for the destructive aim in the total love impulse, including the anger at the frustration which is inevitable because of the omnipotence in the infant's claims" (Winnicott, 1988, p. 86).

EMPATHY

"The state of empathy or being empathic is to perceive the internal frame of reference of another with accuracy and with the emotional components and meanings which pertain thereto as if one were the person, but without ever losing the 'as if' condition. Thus, it means to sense the hurt or the pleasure of another as he senses it and to perceive the causes thereof as he perceives them, but without ever losing the recognition that it is as if I were hurt or pleased and so forth" (Rogers, 1959, pp. 210–211).

FLOW ACTIVITIES

Activities that promote flow are designed to promote the optimal experience. "They have rules that require the learning of skills, they set up goals, they provide feedback, they make control possible. . . . Such *flow activities* have as their primary function the provision of enjoyable experiences" (Csikszentmihalyi, 1990, p. 72).

THREE COMPONENTS OF SELF-IMAGE, OR THE "SELVES" (FRANK, 1958, P. 217)

1. The acting self: The self we present to others that is the total of roles we use to respond in different situations.
2. The perceived self: What I am.
3. The ideal self: What I would like to be or feel I ought to be.

GENUINENESS

According to Rogers (1957/1992), within the realm of the therapeutic relationship, the therapist is a congruent, genuine, and integrated person. "It means that within the relationship he is freely and deeply himself, with his actual experience accurately represented by his awareness of himself. It is the opposite of presenting a façade, either knowingly or unknowingly" (p. 828).

MECHANISMS USED TO MAINTAIN CONSTANCY IN SELF-VIEW IN SPITE OF CONTRARY INFORMATION (FRANK, 1958, P. 220)

- Avoidance: The tendency to avoid experiences that would cause people to change their view of themselves.
- Selective inattention: Not attending to aspects of situations that differ from a person's constancy.
- Self-fulfilling prophecy: Acting in a way to elicit behavior from others that confirms a person's self-picture.

GOOD-ENOUGH MOTHER

Creates a facilitating environment that provides (1) holding, (2) handling, and (3) object presenting (Winnicott, 1965, p. 18).

HOLDING

In the analytic hour, holding is a communication that meets the patient in a short or even momentary point of regression. Winnicott (1972) derived his technique by presenting himself as a process like the mother and infant working through and beyond the "depressive position." In the former process, the child is held by the mother, held over the consequences of the instinctual experience of the infant's integration to bring under control coexisting feelings of love and hate. As Winnicott explains, "I would say that *in the withdrawn state a patient is holding the self* and that if immediately the withdrawn state appears *the analyst can hold the patient*, then what would otherwise have been a withdrawal state becomes a regression. The advantage of regression is that it carries with it the opportunity for correction of inadequate adaptation-to-need in the past history of the patient, that is to say, in the patient's infancy management. By contrast the *withdrawn* state is not profitable and when the patient recovers from a withdrawn state he or she is not changed" (p. 192).

INSTINCT

"Instinct is the term given to powerful biological drives which come and go in the life of the infant or child, and which demand action. The stirrings of instinct cause the child, like any other animal, to make preparations for satisfaction of the full-blown instinct when it eventually reaches a climax of demand. If satisfaction can be provided at the climax of demand, then there is a reward of pleasure and also a temporary relief from instinct. Incomplete or ill-timed satisfaction results in incomplete relief, discomfort, and an absence of a much-needed resting period between waves of demand" (Winnicott, 1988, p. 39).

OCCUPATIONAL BEHAVIOR

"Play, in a chronological or longitudinal sense, we believe, is the antecedent preparation area for work. In a cross-sectional sense we have found it clinically useful to see an adult social-recreation pattern of behavior as a sublatent support to a work pattern. The entire developmental continuum of play and work we designate as occupational behavior" (Reilly, 1969, p. 302).

SEPARATION-INDIVIDUATION PROCESS

"The establishment of a sense of separateness from, and relation to, a world of reality, particularly with regard to the experiences of *one's own body* and to the principal representative of the world as the infant experiences it, the *primary love object*" (Mahler, Pine, & Bergman, 1975, p. 3). The achievements of this phase take place between the fourth or fifth month and the thirtieth or thirty-sixth month.

TRANSFERENCE REACTION

Reacting to someone in the present as if he or she were a significant person in the past (Frank, 1958).

TRANSITIONAL OBJECTS

According to Winnicott (1965, pp. 143–144) these are objects that enable the child to tolerate the frustrations and deprivations of new situations, transitions. They are "the intermediate area of experience, between the thumb and the teddy bear, between the oral erotism and the true object-relationship, between primary creative activity and projection of what has already been introjected" (Winnicott, 1971, p. 2). Winnicott explains that the object may be something like a doll or a teddy bear, probably one particular one that is soft and was introduced to the infant at around ten to twelve months. The object is treated both lovingly and brutally. This is the object that the child would not be separated from when going to bed or one to ever be left behind. "This is a continuation forward of the initial task which the ordinary mother enables her infant to undertake, when by a most delicate active adaptation she offers herself, perhaps her breast, a thousand times at the moment that the baby is ready to create something like the breast that she offers" (p. 144).

THE BORROWED PRACTICE

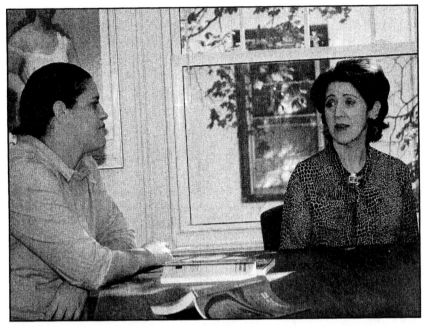

FIGURE 2.1   Building an Alliance through Active Listening, Empathy, and Being Genuine

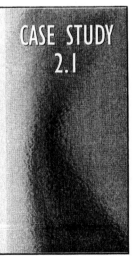

MR. RABINOVICH

CASE STUDY 2.1

*M*r. **Rabinovich,** a retired dentist, now eighty years old, arrived from Russia fifteen years ago. He lives in Boston around the corner from his adult daughter and her husband and their eighteen year-old son. An active and sociable man, Mr. Rabinovich has relied little on others since his wife's death five years ago. While rushing to the Russian restaurant for a birthday celebration, he was run over by a car as he was crossing the street. He sustained a severe head injury and was in a coma. The occupational therapist meets Mr. Rabinovich in the hand clinic several months after the accident. Mr. Rabinovich appears agitated and confused and has memory problems. His daughter speaks for him, although he is able to communicate with some English.

OVERVIEW

*T*he previous chapter explained the philosophical underpinnings of interactive reasoning in occupational therapy. The beliefs borrowed from philosophy and psychology as well as the field itself were reviewed.

This chapter details strategies long used in occupational therapy that are borrowed from other disciplines. Skills and examples from practice include (1) active listening, (2) being genuine and empathic, (3) building an alliance, (4) observing cues and clarifying meaning, (5) giving and receiving information, and (6) reality testing.

NATURE OF EFFECTIVE INTERACTION, COMMUNICATION, AND HELPING

Occupational therapists have borrowed therapeutic strategies from other disciplines that are traditionally known for their approaches to the client and therapist relationship. The perspectives cut across a variety of schools of thought. They include representation from psychodynamic approaches to humanistic, experiential, psychotherapy, and cognitive behavioral counseling techniques (Duncombe, Howe, & Schwartzberg, 1988; Schwartzberg, 1993). The strategies highlighted here are those that pay particular attention to an integrated, client-centered approach. The strategies are congruent with the profession's philosophical and psychological roots. (See Information Checkpoint 2.1.) The reader will see a natural and strong resemblance between the borrowed practice and the philosophical foundations as discussed in chapter 1. It is vital and expected that practice be understood from a cross-cultural perspective. Nowhere is it more important that a person's cultural orientation be taken into account than in the therapist's interactive reasoning. (See Critical Case Question 2.1.) In the opening case, the client's daughter is an essential player in building an alliance with the client. Regardless of his functional problems, for the daughter, it is culturally her role to ensure Mr. Rabinovich's proper care. With or without an interpreter, the daughter is the translator of culture and meaning in the family.

BORROWED STRATEGIES

THE USE OF SELF

The strategies described are not an exhaustive list or description. (See Information Checkpoint 2.2.) This book is a guide to help therapists think about ways of communicating in a therapeutic manner. The strategies are not used in isolation. They are incorporated into the therapist's actions along with the interactive reasoning process. The unique manner in which occupational therapists reason and interact with their clients is given in detail in the chapters that follow. The latter material is presented in the context of settings and populations. This section includes a sample of generic strategies. They are not mutually exclusive categories but rather are related practices. Again, the focus on group work in occupational therapy while very important is not specifically addressed in the strategies described here.

Active Listening: Verbal and Nonverbal Communication

Listening is a very active process that involves observation of verbal and nonverbal communication. The communication imparts both latent and manifest content. The therapist listens to the person with an ear to understanding the story and unfolding narrative. Rather than interpret or direct, the active listener pays attention to the speaker's cues. The therapist's job is to facilitate the flow of communication that is internally motivated by the speaker. In active listening, the therapist also validates the person as the meaning and content come forth. The process of validation is developmental. It starts with "letting the person know" he or she is being heard, accepted, and understood. If the therapeutic relationship is an extended one, in the latter stages, active listening may involve reflecting back themes to the person that have more of an interpretive flavor. Linehan (1997) describes six levels of validation. She points out that the beginning levels are similar to empathy, middle levels empathic interpretation, and the final levels justifying the person as is. (See Information Checkpoint 2.3.) In validating Mr. Rabinovich, regardless of the family's point in the process, his role as elder and prior status as professional need to be acknowledged in interacting with the daughter.

Active listening in a group format requires paying attention to the individual, subgroups, and the group as a whole. As in one-to-one therapeutic relationships, what is being said in a group operates at the latent and manifest levels. Nitsun (1996) identifies several destructive forces in groups that he labels the "antigroup." These forces, if the therapist is unaware of them, can threaten or even destroy a therapeutic or training group. They can also be harnessed to bring forth a group's creative potential. The anti-group, Nitsun explains, is not static, but rather it envelops processes that occur in all groups both natural and therapeutic.

In active listening the therapist is looking for the "direct or more easily discernable" and the "submerged or indirect manifestations" of the process. (See Critical Case Question 2.2.) Nitsun explains that at the manifest level this may be a fear or dislike of groups or actual negative experience in the group itself. The latent or "submerged anti-group attitudes" may be an unconscious or preconscious interpersonal or intrapsychic conflict, often of familial origin, that creates the mistrust of the group. The latent anti-group may remain submerged or may emerge particularly when there is a shared group fantasy about the group and a situation triggers its overt expression. An individual or a subgroup can also be representing the anti-group for the rest of the group. (See Information Checkpoint 2.4.)

Nitsun also explains that the latent and manifest anti-groups feed into each other in a circular fashion. The latent group stimulates disruptions in the manifest group process that then reinforce underlying latent anti-group fantasies. When the therapist actively hears and is aware of these manifestations, the therapeutic potential of the group can be enhanced. In contrast, when the therapist is not listening or cannot hear because of countertransference, then the group can be disruptive or even destroyed.

The techniques used in individual and group intervention vary and will now be described. It is important to understand that these borrowed strategies are combined with occupational therapist's unique methods. Further, there is not always agreement upon the degree to which any of these techniques are successful; for example, information or advice giving and clarifying meaning, also called interpretation.

Being Genuine and Empathic: Establishing Rapport

Borrowing from the humanistic psychologists such as Carl Rogers, as discussed in chapter 1, occupational therapists try to be "genuine" (Rogers, 1957/1992) and "empathic" (Rogers, 1959) with their clients. This involves both sensing and listening to the other person's concerns and conveying this understanding. To accomplish this, therapists must be aware of their own concerns to both distinguish them from others and understand reactions that occur in relating to the client or family member. The degree of genuineness is tempered. The therapist must ask, What will be useful for the person to know as it relates to the therapeutic aims?

The term *genuineness* is similar to more recent relational models of development and therapy that support the notion of emotional connection through mutual empathy (Jordan, Kaplan, Miller, Stiver, & Surrey, 1991). "In mutual empathy one gets to experience oneself as affecting and being affected by another. When one feels empathy from the other person, it provides a palpable sense that one influences and emotionally touches the other person" (Jordan, 1997, p. 343). (See Information Checkpoint 2.5.) Occupational therapists build upon this genuineness with the use of personal stories and metaphors (Borg & Bruce, 1997; Fazio, 1992; Mattingly & Fleming, 1994). This is elaborated on in chapter 3.

Building an Alliance: Communicating with Cultural Sensitivity

Before any therapeutic work can occur, the therapist needs an alliance with the client, student, or significant others. The strength of an alliance builds over time. To build an alliance, the therapist becomes an envelope or a neutral container for the person's affect. That is not to say the therapist does not have feelings or reactions. Rather, the therapist ideally and necessarily must be conscious of these feelings and not act upon them. Therapists suspend their own needs and provide what is necessary for the client to feel safe. Needless to say, this must occur within appropriate professional boundaries. Nevertheless, with short-term interventions, the connection must be made immediately. The therapist's task is to convey interest in the person. Helpees must be convinced that they are understood and that their wishes are taken into account. Being honest about the purpose and nature of the relationship is critical. When the therapist is of a different cultural background from the other person building an alliance may be more difficult. It requires learning about the other's culture from his or her perspective and not imposing one's own values. (See Critical Case Question 2.3.)

Observing Cues and Clarifying Meaning: Stages of Effective Helping

There are cues that are both verbal and nonverbal, and as mentioned earlier, both manifest and latent. The therapist can clarify meaning by asking directly or indirectly for further information. Egan (1982) has identified stages in his outline of counseling or effective helping strategies. (See Information Checkpoint 2.6.)

Many others have also described helping strategies for observing cues and clarifying meaning. A main principle is that the counseling relationship is a developmental process. The process of problem exploration and clarification is appropriate after "attending" and "actively listening" to the client's concerns (Egan, 1982). As the relationship builds trust, themes can be explored and elaborated on in greater depth. Regrettably, under current systems of service delivery in settings such as the inpatient and outpatient hospital, such relationships are curtailed, the goals more short term, and the intervention aimed at discharge environments. This requires that the intervention goals and strategies be different from those in more long-term settings. It is also important to recognize differences in what is possible in community and prevention programs versus those directed at altering pathology or performance components such as the skills underlying occupational capacity. Further, as discussed previously, when working with groups the therapist is wise to consider meanings at the level of the individual, subgroups, and the group as a whole.

Giving and Receiving Information

Strategies for giving and receiving information are derived from therapists' perceptions of their role. The therapist can act as teacher, advisor, counselor, or aide. In all instances, the offering of advice should also be questioned as a viable method. It is more profitable to consider two questions:

1. Under what conditions should the information be given?
2. What type of information can be processed and integrated?

The timing and relevance of information are essential to its meaning to the client or student as well as to those significant in life such as partners and family members, employers, and teachers. For the Rabinoviches, education is essential to their understanding of the head injury, its sequel, and short- and long-term goals of occupational therapy.

Reality Testing: Empowerment through Validation

This complicated strategy is hard to explain. The therapist both becomes a mirror and forms a boundary. The act of reality testing involves reflecting back the multivaried senses and perceptions to restore or create a wholeness rather than a state of vulnerability. It involves framing for the first time or reframing an idea to make it coherent within a larger picture. The therapist may need to reality test with the person for several reasons. The foremost reason is to protect the safety of individuals if their judgement is impaired by the absence of this capability. (See Critical Case Question 2.4.)

In reality testing, the therapist is empathic and validating. In her explanation of the differences between validation and empathy Linehan (1997) points out that in the former a conclusion is made about what is being presented or the behavior or experience. She observes that "although empathy is necessary for clinical validation, it is not sufficient. Needed in addition is an analysis of the client's response in light of its relationship to context (i.e., the empirical situation) and its function (i.e., as a means to an end)" (p. 360). Linehan's model is useful for gauging the degrees of empathy and validation. (See Information Checkpoint 2.7.)

BACK TO MR. RABINOVICH

In building a relationship with Mr. Rabinovich, the occupational therapist worked with both him and his daughter. Through active listening the therapist learned that the client had been quite withdrawn before his accident and highly distracted. His daughter at first denied the possibility that her father was depressed at the time. Eventually, the daughter accepted that her father's loss of family, friends, occupation, country, and social status, and thus his psychological state and social well-being, was significantly related to his physical well-being. Once the daughter's needs and role were validated, the therapy progressed and Mr. Rabinovich actively participated in his occupational therapy program and after-care follow-up plan.

SUMMARY

The theory and strategies borrowed from other fields were explained. The techniques overlap, as can be expected in interactions that are process oriented. Following the philosophical assumptions and reasoning borrowed, one can see a direct progression to the thinking and practice of occupational therapists. These ideas are discussed in chapter 3, where the derived occupational therapy practice is presented.

REFLECTIVE QUESTIONS

- What happens in active listening? Think about a situation where you felt someone truly listened to you or others. Describe the nature of your experience and what the other person did, said, or did not do or say. Was the experience consistent with active listening? If not, describe how it significantly differed.
- How are the latent and manifest issues expressed in a group situation? Reflecting upon your own experience in a therapy group or other small group, describe an issue that emerged as a pattern. What themes and issues discussed or not discussed may have been related and left unexplored?
- What are essential actions on the therapist's part when building an alliance and trust? Reflect upon your own experience where you trusted another individual. What actions built that trust?
- How is empathy conveyed, and how can it differ from validation?
- Describe how you imagine the progression of working with someone from the beginning stages of therapy to the latter, more advanced stages. How do these stages differ, and what line of reasoning would you use at each stage, and why? Reflect upon aspects of the developing relationship that would be more difficult for you and describe why.

INFORMATION CHECKPOINTS

2.1. HUMANISTIC PHILOSOPHY IN OCCUPATIONAL THERAPY (BORG & BRUCE, 1997)

- Motivation exists within individuals.
- The healthy need for autonomy is innate.
- Each person lives in a daily world that is self-perceived.
- To be meaningful, the experience of occupational therapy must be perceived as relevant to the person.
- Optimum function occurs when the individual experiences self-comfort, is open, is guided by his or her own beliefs and values, and uses skills and abilities to the fullest possible to do tasks that are valued while respecting others' needs and rights.
- Successful intervention requires that the occupation be valued and meaningful to facilitate a context for change from within the individual.

2.2. THE BORROWED PRACTICE

- Active listening
- Being genuine and empathic
- Building an alliance
- Observing cues and clarifying meaning
- Giving and receiving information
- Reality testing

2.3. LEVELS OF VALIDATION (LINEHAN, 1997)

- Level 1: Listening and observing
- Level 2: Accurate reflection
- Level 3: Articulating the unverbalized
- Level 4: Validating in terms of sufficient but not necessarily valid causes
- Level 5: Validating as reasonable in the moment
- Level 6: Treating the person as valid—radical genuineness

2.4. ANTI-GROUP

The anti-group manifests itself in different ways. Therapists should recognize the various expressions to positively influence group process. The dimensions of anti-group include the following (Nitsun, 1996, p. 57):

- Degree of overt versus covert expression of anti-group tendencies
- Influence of the group's stage of development on anti-group tendencies
- Indirect and symbolic expressions of the anti-group
- Transformation of the anti-group into a positive, constructive group force

2.5. EMPATHY

"Empathy involves the capacity to perceive another's affective state, to resonate with that emotional state, and to gain some understanding or clarity about the other's subjective world. Rather than a more distance-mediated way of knowing through cognitive channels alone, empathy involves an emotional resonance that gives one a compelling psychological-physiological sense of joining with the experience of another person" (Jordan, 1997, p. 344).

2.6. STAGES AND RELATED SKILLS OF EFFECTIVE HELPING (EGAN, 1982)

STAGE I: PROBLEM EXPLORATION AND CLARIFICATION

- Attending and active listening
- Accurate empathy
- Using probes in problem exploration and definition
- Respect, genuineness, and social influence

STAGE II: DEVELOPING NEW PERSPECTIVES AND SETTING GOALS

- Summarizing, information giving, and advanced empathy
- Confrontation, counselor self-sharing, and skills of immediacy
- Setting problem-managing goals

STAGE III: ACTION

Development and sequencing of programs

- Helping clients identify program possibilities
- Helping clients choose programs
- Helping clients order program steps

Implementing and evaluating programs

- Helping clients implement programs: Skills and strategies
- Helping clients evaluate the helping process

2.7. DEVELOPMENTAL STEPS IN VALIDATION (LINEHAN, 1997)

Based upon Linehan's scheme, therapists can ask the following questions:

- Step 1: What is the client saying, feeling, and doing?
- Step 2: Am I accurately reflecting back the client's own feelings, thoughts, assumptions, and behaviors?
- Step 3: Have I validly "read" the client's behavior and conveyed my understanding of events not directly communicated?
- Step 4: Have I communicated that the client's behavior is understandable and justifiable in light of the relevant causes?
- Step 5: Have I told the client that in terms of the client's normative biological functioning, current events, and life goals the behavior is justified and reasonable?
- Step 6: Have I recognized the client's strengths while maintaining an empathic understanding of the person's actual difficulties and incapacities?

CRITICAL CASE QUESTIONS

2.1. As a therapist, you know a few things about Mr. Rabinovich. What are known aspects of his cultural orientation? What more would you like to know about his culture and its meaning?

2.2. Speculate on what might be some direct or manifest concerns and indirect or latent concerns of Mr. Rabinovich and his daughter. What are they, and how might they be expressed?

2.3. In building an alliance, what roles would you assume with Mr. Rabinovich and his daughter?

2.4. What dilemmas might you encounter in reality testing with Mr. Rabinovich about his current circumstance? How would you intervene? What is the daughter's role in the process?

KEY TERMS

ACCURATE EMPATHY

"Helpers are accurately empathic if they can (1) get inside their client's world, get a feeling for what this world is like, and look at the outer world through their client's perspective or frame of reference and . . . (2) communicate this understanding in a way that shows they have some understanding of their client's feelings and the experiences and behaviors to which these feelings relate" (Egan, 1982, p. 86).

ACTIVE LISTENING

"Total or complete listening [active listening] involves two things; first, observing and interpreting the client's nonverbal behavior—posture, facial expressions, movement, tone of voice, and the like—and, second, listening to and interpreting the client's verbal messages" (Egan, 1982, p. 63).

ADVANCED ACCURATE EMPATHY

Based upon client cues, the helper communicates what the client says indirectly by implication and hints as well as what is said nonverbally (Egan, 1982, p. 40).

THE ANTI-GROUP

The anti-group is a construct that Nitsun (1996) created to describe destructive forces that threaten to destroy a group (pp. 1–2). The following are sources of these destructive processes:

- Underlying fear, anxiety, and distrust of the group process rather than experiencing the group as an "empathic mirror" of understanding.
- Frustration of "narcissistic needs" and experiencing the group as depriving, neglectful, and undermining.
- Inability to contain and resolve direct confrontation between members or indirect expressions of aggression such as envy, rivalry, or destructive competition, causing the group to feel unsafe.

ATTENDING

Helpers letting clients know they are with them and completely available to them at the time of helping by behaviors such as making eye contact and avoiding distracting behaviors (Egan, 1982, p. 35).

CONFRONTATION

Challenging discrepancies, distortions, games, and smoke screens in client's life and in relationship with the helper so that it leads to self-understanding and constructive change (Egan, 1982, p. 40).

CROSS-CULTURAL PERSPECTIVE

Consideration is given to cultural orientation in the understanding and manner in which the therapist thinks about and carries out any intervention. Culture includes a person's sexual, religious, spiritual, and socioeconomic orientations as well as those of their family, community, and other significant institutions and relationships.

COUNTERTRANSFERENCE

The therapist's own reactions, his or her thoughts and feelings, conscious, preconscious, or unconscious.

GENUINENESS

Genuineness involves the helper's refusing to overemphasize his or her role, being spontaneous, avoiding defensiveness, being consistent, and being open (Egan, 1982, pp. 127–131).

IMMEDIACY

Encouraging direct, mutual talk and exploring the here and now of client-helper interactions so that clients get a better picture of their interpersonal style (Egan, 1982, p. 40).

LATENT CONTENT

Latent content refers to things that are not said and may be outside the person's own awareness.

MANIFEST CONTENT

Manifest content refers to what is said and consciously understood by the speaker.

PRECONSCIOUS THOUGHTS

These are thoughts, feelings, fantasies, and so forth that are not readily within a person's conscious awareness but are available to the person. Unconscious thoughts are those unavailable without analysis of dreams, symbolism, and free associations as done in psychoanalysis.

PROBES

"Probes are ways of helping a client articulate a problem situation in more specific and concrete terms" (Egan, 1982, p. 36).

REALITY

There are several ways to define reality, depending upon one's theoretical perspective. From a purely philosophical framework, one can take the existential stance that reality is in the perception of the individual. Alternatively, one can say that it is the person's way of knowing or thinking. Borrowing from psychology, perceiving reality can be viewed as a function of one's ego. With a neurological perspective, the perception of reality is one of the executive functions of the brain. For our purposes, reality is all of the former. Reality is multidetermined. It is not one thing.

SOCIAL INFLUENCE

Perceived, positive attractiveness of the helper, such as being trustworthy and competent (Egan, 1982).

THE OCCUPATIONAL THERAPY PRACTICE

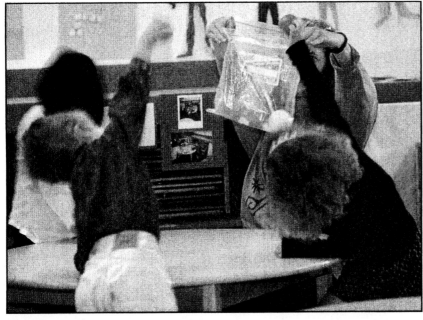

FIGURE 3.1 Active Participation through Occupation-Based Meaning and Match

MRS. SMITH

CASE STUDY
3.1

*M*rs. Smith is a retired art teacher living in the suburbs with her son and his young family. Having smoked for over forty-five years, she was recently hospitalized for chronic obstructive pulmonary disease. The occupational therapist anticipates that Mrs. Smith will have difficulty resuming her former role of caring for her grandchildren. This is the first day of outpatient therapy. Mrs. Smith appears tense and smells of cigarette smoke. She greets the therapist warmly but cautions there is little time for the appointment. Her son is already late for work. It is mid-July, and the weather has been unusually hot for several weeks.

OVERVIEW

*T*he **prior** chapter explained occupational therapy from the perspective of ideas borrowed from other fields and outlined strategies and skills for engaging in a therapeutic relationship. These strategies and skills included (a) active listening, (b) being genuine and empathic, (c) building an alliance, (d) observing cues and clarifying meaning, (e) giving and receiving information, and (f) reality testing.

The occupational therapist also employs a unique set of ideas and means of practice. This point of view is foremost differentiated by its philosophy as a phenomenological practice as detailed in chapter 1. Current occupational therapy practice, presented in this chapter, concludes the introductory part of this book. Chapter 3 begins with the case study of Mrs. Smith, an individual with problems typically seen by occupational therapists. Reflecting on Mrs. Smith's situation provides an illustration of reasoning in practice. Models and strategies that pertain to interactive aspects of the client-centered practice and the client-therapist relationship in occupational therapy are presented. The strategies selected reflect those reported in the literature and found in the author interviews of therapists. (See Information Checkpoint 3.1.)

A strong relationship exists between the themes and techniques derived from the interviews. (See Table 3.1.) The techniques clearly match what therapists report about their approach to interactive reasoning in occupational therapy. Although there might be slight differences in emphasis between settings and populations, the therapists' perspectives were all quite similar.

Recently there has been a renewed interest in occupational therapy models that pertain to interactive aspects of the client-centered practice (Law, 1998; Lawlor & Mattingly, 1998) and the client-therapist relationship in occupational therapy (Borg & Bruce, 1997; Davidson & Peloquin, 1998; Norrby & Bellner, 1995; Peloquin, 1998; Rosa & Hasselkus, 1996). The perspective presented here

TABLE 3.1
THEMES AND TECHNIQUES OF INTERACTIVE REASONING IN OCCUPATIONAL THERAPY

INTERVIEW-GENERATED THEMES

Active participation and collaboration
Engaging/connecting and creating a holding environment
Exploring/interpreting motives as well as occupation-based meanings
Listening
Understanding and use of narrative/symbolic

TECHNIQUES CHARACTERISTIC OF PRACTICE

Selling
Giving back
Engaging the mood
Validating
Holding

is drawn primarily from Fleming and Mattingly's (1994) model of clinical reasoning as well as from related research of occupational therapists and the students and faculty at Tufts University. Emphasis is given to the themes identified by the author's research. These themes are further described in Part II—The Practice Environments—and Part III—The Practice Populations.

MODES OF REASONING

Occupational therapists come to understand the client as a person through multiple modes of reasoning (Fleming, 1994). As Fleming and Mattingly (2000) state, "Action is both a concrete event and a reasoning strategy that mediates the flow of therapy from image to result" (p. 55). They further explain that much of this knowledge is both "professional knowledge" and "tacit knowledge." Tacit knowledge is based on the therapist's experience. It is called into action but is not necessarily cognitively focused at a conscious level. As Mattingly (1991a) early on explained, in occupational therapy, clinical reasoning is based upon tacit understanding and habitual knowledge that is experienced based. Fleming (1991b) coined the phrase "the three-track mind" to represent the types of reasoning used by therapists in their daily practice. She called them "procedural reasoning," "interactive reasoning," and "conditional reasoning."

Much work has been completed since Mattingly and Fleming's original study (Mattingly & Gillette, 1991). A variety of images have been used to describe clinical reasoning in occupational therapy (Crabtree, 1998). It is now widely accepted that occupational therapists employ five types of reasoning, as summarized by Neistadt (1998): (1) narrative reasoning, (2) procedural reasoning, (3) interactive reasoning, (4) pragmatic reasoning, and (5) conditional reasoning. (See Key Terms for definitions.)

According to Neistadt (1998), "Interactive reasoning yields an understanding of what the disease or disability means to the client (i.e., the client's illness experience). Interactive reasoning also encompasses the interpersonal interactions between therapists and clients" (p. 229). The primary aim here is to explain interactive reasoning—the thoughts and means used by an occupational therapist to get to know a person and engage the intervention process. However, to truly understand the occupational therapist's perspective, the other types of reasoning must also be understood and applied in relation to each other.

STRATEGIES REPORTED IN THE OCCUPATIONAL THERAPY LITERATURE

The occupational therapist understands the meaning of occupational performance problems from the client's perspective (Crepeau, 1991; Fleming, 1991a, 1991b, 1993; Schell & Cervero, 1993). Strategies employed in this therapeutic relationship include narrative thinking and critical discourse with clients (Cohn, 1989, 1991; Fleming, 1991a, 1991b; Mattingly, 1991a, 1991b; Mostert, Zacharkiewicz, & Fossey, 1996; Price-Lackey & Cashman, 1996). Some other occupational therapy strategies reported in the literature include but are not limited to the following:

- Communicating a sense of trust, hope (Langthaler, 1990; Spencer, Davidson, & White, 1997), and empathy (Peloquin, 1995).
- Encouraging collaboration by creating choices, individualizing treatment, structuring success, "doing" for clients and "doing" for therapists within professional boundaries, and joint problem solving (Mattingly & Fleming, 1994).
- Interpreting motives and meanings from cues based on what clients do and say (Mattingly & Fleming, 1994; Sviden & Saljo, 1993).
- Reasoning and acting through empathy toward the client, active listening, values clarification, affirmation of the client, nonreaction to expressed poor judgement, and goal setting (Bradburn, 1992), and understanding visions and images (Peloquin, 1995).
- Using life histories, metaphors, story making, and storytelling (Borg & Bruce, 1997; Clark, 1993; Fazio, 1992; Frank, 1996; Mattingly, 1991b; Price-Lackey & Cashman, 1996), anchoring, and metaphorical directives.
- In a group, communicating and considering the perspectives of the individual and the group as a whole (Howe & Schwartzberg, 1995, 2001).

RECENT PERSPECTIVES FROM OCCUPATIONAL THERAPY PRACTITIONERS

During the course of writing this book, the author conducted thirty-nine interviews with therapists from a variety of settings in the Greater Boston area. The purpose of the interviews was twofold. First, the author wanted to hear directly from therapists about their perceptions of interactive reasoning in occupational therapy. Second, based on these first-hand accounts, the literature could be evaluated in terms of its validity and completeness.

The respondents were both novice and seasoned practitioners, including some administrators and faculty with considerable clinical experience. They were selected in consultation with the researcher's colleagues, through respondent referral, and by word of mouth. Not one therapist refused to be interviewed. The therapists were asked to respond to two main questions:

1. What would you consider the elements of best interactive practice?
2. What would you consider the elements of reasoning in this type of practice?

The interviews were conducted both by telephone and in the practice setting. They were limited to thirty minutes, and verbatim notes were taken. Common themes and techniques were then identified through an analysis of the transcriptions.

THEMES

Five themes were identified: (1) active participation and collaboration, (2) engaging/connecting with the person and creating a holding environment, (3) exploring and interpreting motives as well as occupation-based meanings, (4) listening, and (5) understanding and use of narrative/symbolic. (See Information Checkpoint 3.2.)

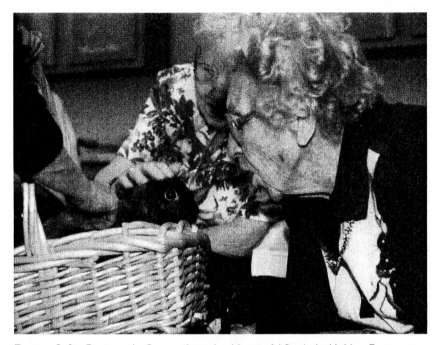

FIGURE 3.2   Engaging the Person through a Meaningful Symbolic Holding Environment

Active Participation and Collaboration

Therapists used the following concepts to guide their interactions with clients. In particular, the methods were used to elicit each client's active participation and collaboration. They included offering control by creating choices, being client centered, explaining the role of occupational therapy, helping the client to develop insight into problems with functioning, and joint problem solving.

As the chapter opening case study and the following examples demonstrate, a collaborative relationship is a necessary condition for the tasks of occupational therapy. Mrs. Smith has a powerful addiction. She values her role as caretaker and loves her family. Her pulmonary-respiratory disease has severely affected her functioning and required hospitalization. Regardless of these factors, without the client—and perhaps family—involvement in the process, the intervention is doomed and Mrs. Smith's functioning will deteriorate as she conceals her smoking habit.

Offering Control by Creating Choices

Therapists try to give clients choices whenever possible. They believe that having choice offers clients a degree of control that is often lacking. The loss of control is viewed as being due to the confinements of hospitalization, change in function, and loss of former occupational roles. As Rebecca Reynolds, OTR/L, private practitioner and founder of the Concord Seabury School, puts it, "I try to be conscious of coming in with the knowledge that being in a hospital bed is a very disempowered position. . . . I found the hardest thing of being in a hospital is watching the person being stripped of his or her control. I would like to make sure there is a moment of connection and problem solving. . . . Making resources available where people can find interest in their own learning and taking control." With sarcasm Jim Sellers, OTR/L, of New England Sinai Hospital and Rehabilitation Center, further points out that hospitals are confining places yet there is pressure not to duplicate services. He says, " I always try to think about the elements of choice and control. Especially in a hospital, there is little choice and control. We don't want to duplicate services!"

Client-Centered Approach

Evaluate Client's Response

Therapists repeatedly mention a client-centered approach as central to occupational therapy. They define this as eliciting the client in treatment planning from the point of evaluation through termination. Families and significant others are often included in this client-centered process. They are enlisted to both authenticate the situation and add clarity to the picture of the person's functioning. Although therapists believe in this approach, they also surmise that at some level there are those therapists who do not trust it. Jim Sellers points out the irony that clients do not trust a prefabricated approach. He candidly states, "You must start with the person, with what really means something to someone. The rest, the range of motion, the endurance, will follow. I believe people really do not trust this approach. They go for *component land.* They use a checklist and get information they may not necessarily need because it is on the form. I try to find out what does the patient need the most."

Select and Use Activities As Well As Context

Another part of being client-centered is finding activities that are meaningful to the person. Norrby and Bellner (1995) concur that "in order to carry out the work of occupational therapy, the therapist enters more fully into the client's situation by focusing on the key needs or problems as perceived by the client himself" (p. 44). Kristina Dulberger, OTR/L, of the Perkins School for the Blind, captures this theme when she speaks about setting up the environment to compensate for the impairment. She puts it, "You try to find meaningful activities that are a success. That is the just right challenge. You adapt the activities and the materials so the activity is a success. Picking the 'just right challenge' is also my challenge."

Finding meaningful activities requires the therapist to analyze the activity component demands and take into account past successes. Therapists use a variety of theories to make decisions about how to modify the environment or interaction. Dulburger works with students who are deaf and blind. Her clinical decisions are often made based on her knowledge of the children's sensory processing. She gives an example: "If a student becomes overwhelmed by sensory stimuli, then I would modify the environment and task to the optimal level for attention." She further explains, "Depending on the student, it would be whatever the condition is that affects the treatment; for example, if hypotonicity affected performance, then I would want the student sitting in an optimal supported seating, if that was what I happened to be working on." Her examples always come back to the recurrent theme of the spontaneity required. Interactive reasoning is a mental exercise that quickly moves between observation and action. Such spontaneity is further described later in the chapter in the section on "listening" in the "moment to moment."

Role of Occupational Therapy

Occupational therapists see it as essential that the client first have a clear idea of what the profession is about. As Sherlyn Fenton, OTR/L, of St. Camillus Health Center and Hospice, explains, "The client should be getting good descriptions of what is to be expected in OT. What are we expecting by the approach? There should be a clear definition of the role of OT, the participation expected of the client, and what would be the expected or desired outcomes." According to Pat Keck, OTR/L, of Beth Israel Deaconess Medical Center in Boston, and a seasoned therapist of thirty years, part of showing dignity and respect for the client occurs during the first few moments, starting with immediately explaining the role of occupational therapy and going into what is important to the client. Other therapists report, in addition to what the client finds interesting and valuable, describing information and an explanation of treatment goals as important motivational strategies (Norrby & Bellner, 1995).

Client Insight into Impact on Function

Many therapists explain that an important part of their role is helping the client to understand the disease process and its impact on the person's routine. For many clients this is a difficult task in itself because of communication problems, cognitive impairments in ability to think abstractly, denial, lack of information, and the like. Michael Davison, OTR/L, of the New England Sinai Hospital and Rehabilitation Center suggests that those clients who say they do not know ask, "Did you ever know anyone with this problem? How did it affect them?" The client's insight is not limited to working with adults. Sharon Ray, OTR/L, of Tufts University, Boston School of Occupational Therapy, is particularly sensitive to the self-esteem issues involved with children. She explains the motives for her actions as, "I try to follow the child's cues. As [children get] older, they may self-identify. As they ask, I give more information. I try being where the children are—tying my actions with the usual—because otherwise they think he or she is bad." For the child, being perceived and treated as different, not usual, may contribute to thinking he or she is bad. As Norrby and Bellner (1995) report, "Helping clients adapt to reality is built on real situations in every-day actions which the client has to handle in his every-day life" (p. 44).

Such actions require the therapist to employ diagnostic and hypothetical reasoning. The occupational therapy diagnosis is derived from cue acquisition, hypothesis generation, cue interpretation, and hypothesis evaluation. Through the former, the therapist creates a clinical image of the impact of diagnostically related problems on occupational deficits in terms of performance components and occupation role performance (Rogers & Holm, 1991). Fleming (1991a) points out such hypothetical reasoning involves application of a scientific model similarly used in medicine.

The case of Mrs. Smith is a good example of the impact of denial in the face of information. The client "knew" the facts of her medical condition. It was only when she could no longer get out of bed to answer the door for her grandchildren did she have insight about the impact of her disease on her daily functioning.

Joint Problem Solving

Therapists value problem solving with the client to the fullest capacity possible. By encouraging the client to buy into the plan, joint problem solving is possible.

Mattingly and Fleming (1994a) found joint problem solving a commonly used strategy among occupational therapists for developing cooperation. Once Mrs. Smith acknowledged her condition, she was then able to accept her son's home as her own and with her occupational therapist plan strategies for energy conservation and smoking cessation.

Engaging/Connecting and Creating a Holding Environment

Connecting with the person means the therapist must establish trust. This is conveyed through being empathic and truly showing regard for the person. Strategies are used to adapt to the individual in terms of personality, behavior, emotional needs, and functional level (Norrby & Bellner, 1995). The therapist uses the following approaches to engage with the client: establishing trust, conveying hope, being empathic, and demonstrating regard for the individual.

Trust

Therapists use many strategies for facilitating trust with the client. This may entail the therapist's taking time to validate his or her understanding of the client's perception of the situation. "There is a trust in the client, in the therapist," says Regina Doherty, OTR/L, of Massachusetts General Hospital. A big part of establishing trust appears to be allowing the person time to express him or herself. As Michael Nardone, OTR/L, of University of Hartford, explains: "One thing that I learned over time was to allow clients to express themselves and for me to be comfortable with silence. It was trying not to rush people. It is allowing people to express themselves and not to push them beyond where they want to go."

Hope

Often the therapist must hold out hope for the client and family. Part of holding out hope is in providing an environment that will allow the person to function at his or her maximum capacity. This may involve using a comforting tone of voice, providing cues, and acting as a memory for the client. Kathy Hanlon, OTR/L, of Newton Wellesley Hospital, is very clear about her approach, explaining it this way: "I will always give hope that they will not always be where they are now. I will always give hope that they will not always feel this way. I might find something related to their occupation that might draw them out if they are withdrawn. Always try to help people look at the hopeful side of things but not in a patronizing kind of way." The sense of hopefulness is related to the importance of the client's active participation. Janet Kahane, OTR/L, also of Newton Wellesley Hospital, explains the connection: "There is the patient's sense of helpfulness and hopefulness on my part. There needs to be something that the client can buy into and wants to work on. . . . Patients have a clear understanding of what we are offering them. This can instill a feeling of 'hopefulness' as the client starts to feel better about an area he/she may have neglected."

Empathy

Empathy is considered an essential tool in client interactions and working with families. It is "the therapist's ability to listen, be attentive and understand the message the client wants to express" (Norrby & Bellner, 1995, p. 43). The skilled therapists are the ones who can empathize in a manner that gives back control to the client. Regina Doherty gives an example of what she might say to a client: "I know you are really frustrated because your arm can't do what you want it to do." She explains her rationale: "The bonding occurs because the client thinks the therapist *really* understands and can help. People feel obligated to accept what is offered them. Information doesn't do anything for them. It really doesn't change the situation. The information is one more thing they have to accept. They don't have control of it. They can't unherniate a disk. By giving choices and by helping them understand how it impacts their function it gives them back control."

Mutual Regard

Mutual regard must be felt. The process of establishing mutual regard is observed to be tricky to describe. When pressed, Dalit Waller, OTR/L, of Neville Manor Nursing Home, elaborates. "The more I understand who the person is, what has meaning to the person, to his or her values, then I try to incorporate those elements. The driving force is to keep people focused to maximize the use of time so that they get things accomplished according to what they want. It is an immediate process of showing regard for the person, like Carl Rogers."

Exploring and Interpreting Motives As Well As Occupation Based Meanings

Exploration involves the individual and, in a therapeutic group, both the individual and the the group as a whole.

The Individual

Select and Use Treatment to Prepare for Engagement in Occupation

Therapists uniformly agree that understanding the person's past roles and interests is essential. Many talk about wanting to get to know the person. Dan Kerls, OTR/L, of Newton Wellesley Hospital, makes it seem simple. He states, "What I do is something in between theory and intuition. After a while it is just in you! When I think about things I learned in school, what comes to my mind are a lot of theories on role, role dysfunction. I see how important patients' roles are to them and then I empathize with them. What is going on is a cross between reality testing, empathy, and looking at what patients value in terms of their role. I am trying to look at the whole picture. I am looking at what the family is doing. Is there going to be support in the community? I ask the people about their past or their hobbies to get a better sense of who they are. Part of this I knew, part of this was learned from mentors, and part of it is learning what is meaningful and having to do that in my occupational therapy class about what was meaningful to me."

The Individual and the Group as a Whole

Most of the therapists addressed interactive reasoning from the perspective of one-to-one relationships. However, groups are widely used in occupational therapy, and the reasoning strategies deserve separate consideration. Mary Barnes, OTR/L, of University of Massachusetts Medical Center and Tufts University, Boston School of Occupational Therapy, says, "The ideal group would need me less. It would be more like a 'mature' group. One can infer when thinking about the individual in the group one needs to take into account the influence of the group's process. There is a dynamic relationship between how the group manages the task or occupation and the individual's adaptation [to the task]."

Listening

Listening is a special skill that involves several strategies, which, for occupational therapists, include active listening, validation and genuineness, affirmation of the client, empathic connection and rapport, goal setting, and being in the moment to moment. These tactics are not discreet categories but overlapping strategies.

Active Listening (Cue Identification)

Deborah Slater, OTR/L, of New England Baptist Hospital, an experienced therapist and administrator, gives clear advice: "Ask only a few questions. Have the right questions and draw people out. That is the main strategy." Asking the right questions is not an easy task, especially for the novice practitioner. After one and a half years of working in early intervention, Laura Snell, OTR/L, of Bay Cove Early Intervention Program, gives some guidelines to enable active listening. She observes: "It is a two-way street. It is not always the way it is told to you. I try to reflect and listen actively. What is the theory telling me? It tells me not to pass judgement and not to really be involved in the conversation. I am trying to help parents get at what they are feeling and reflect what they are saying to help them help themselves." Active listening means therapists must put their own expectations aside. It is clearly not thinking about a body part. As Linda McGettigan, OTR/L, of New England Sinai Hospital and Rehabilitation Center, puts it: "If I go in and think, this patient is a hip and is going to be here two weeks, I am not listening to what the patient wants to achieve." She further explains, "What I am doing is looking for cues from the patient. . . . I am looking for connecting the patient to what we are doing here."

Validation and Genuineness

Validation is viewed as key to therapeutic interaction. The therapist must be open to seeing things from the vantage point of the client, student, family member, and so on. To be successful in this transaction, the therapist must be perceived as being genuine. Ellen Cohen Kaplan, OTR/L, private practitioner associated with Harvard Community Health Plan, strongly believes validation is primary. She states what so many expressed in different words: "The first thing I think is how would I want to make them comfortable. To validate. To echo back. To paraphrase. Empathy is the first rule of thumb. The second thing is that having a real comfort level with the material can let me go into more depth. I am analyzing, using many metacognitive processes, analysis of countertransference. Frame it and state in the moment. Remember that this is not my family member." Cohen Kaplan further explains that connecting with the client is part of conveying unconditional acceptance. "I make a point to connect with people [individually]. I talk to them about things that have nothing to do with the group. The one-to-one connection makes them feel an unconditional acceptance. It can be around anything, for example, sports. The better your fund of knowledge, the more points to connect."

Affirmation of the Client

Affirmation involves relating what is going on in the session to the bigger picture that therapists talk about—occupation. Therapists constantly refer to the importance of relating the session to what is going on outside the session to the person's life.

Empathic Connection and Rapport

Empathy is directly linked with therapist reports of the importance of active listening and, as discussed earlier, validation. This involves what therapists call "looking at the bigger picture." Validation often includes information about the person's family, community, and occupations—past, present, and future. Kathy Hanlon, a highly experienced therapist working in community education, says this about a good empathic connection. "People have a real sense of the client and what the person is going through. The therapist sees the person and not a category." Hanlon goes on to describe what for her "is all happening in a split second."

Hanlon is also cautious about differentiating her own feelings from those of the client. She explains, "Sometimes I use my own feelings. I try to read [my feelings] to see if this is coming from [the client], for example their anxiety, or is the person hitting my buttons. This is all happening in a split second. This quick mental checklist happens in a split second. Do I understand this person's state of mind knowing my state of mind may not be the same? I may understand the feeling state, although I am not feeling it at the time. I am a good picker upper regarding reading a person's affect. It is kind of an intuitive thing. To notice that, not just absorb this. . . . You need to handle the personal reaction and put this aside if it is coming from you. You need to contain it yourself and put it in the background and deal with the client. It needs to be OUT of the interaction." Others in occupational therapy (Norrby & Bellner, 1995) have also reported the important link between empathy and therapists' self-awareness of their own values, feelings, and norms on the helping process.

Goal Setting

Outcomes of Occupational Engagement and Participation

Setting goals involves validating the person's concerns and clarifying them to be sure you are not misunderstanding. Sue Brown, OTR/L, of St. Joseph's Hospital, explains, "I sit at eye level or below. I always try to explain to the best of their understanding what the activity is and try to relate it to their goals. I explain things in relation to the home environment and do this in setting up the treatment."

Moment to Moment

Many therapists found it difficult to name theories that guide their practice. The notion of intuitive response and adapting in the moment better portrays therapists' perceptions of interactions. Sue Brown believes that part of it is intuition and getting to know the client. She cautions repeatedly to take time to look for signals for what works best for the individual, to take a few moments and reflect back what you are hearing in the moment. "It has to be a quick judgement, and I think that any lag time will disrupt that rapport. . . . I believe they give you signals.

And a lot of people miss it! I think you are always observing, analyzing, and reevaluating. You look for what works best for the clients. It may be talking softly. I think it is just a teasing out of different things."

Understanding and Use of Narrative/Symbolic

Occupational therapists are highly skilled at both the analysis and the use of the symbolic in interactions with their clients. Some of the strategies they use include eliciting life history, example by metaphor, storytelling, and verbalizing images. They create a picture of the person's actual and future wishes, needs, resources, and limitations (Norrby & Bellner, 1995). As Mattingly (1998) also observed, "In occupational therapy, transformation and conversion are often metaphorically expressed through the symbol of the journey" (p. 164).

Life History

Therapists use the client's history to get to know the client and to comprehend what is important. This theme cuts across populations and settings. However, therapists in inpatient settings talked most about gathering information about the person's past occupational roles. They also referred to getting to know about the client through cues in the person's room such as family pictures or the absence of such.

The aim of getting life history is linked to the therapist's wish to understand how to motivate the person and engage him or her in the therapy process. For example, one can see a very bold pattern of caretaking in the chapter's opening case study. Mrs. Smith is a retired teacher and cares for her grandchildren. In spite of her discomfort over her son's being late for work, she greets the therapist warmly. Her interaction with the therapist is purportedly aimed to protect the therapist's feelings and appear cooperative. The scenario helps to tell the story of her codependency. Mrs. Smith has a lifelong pattern of caring for others at the expense of her own health and needs. By maintaining this role, while her condition deteriorates, she protects a competing unspoken need to have others take care of her.

Metaphors

Therapists talk about the importance of time and well-chosen interventions. A metaphor can become a way of quickly translating meanings between the therapist and the client or family member. "By definition, a metaphor is a transfer of meaning" (Jones, 1991, p. 30). "Metaphorical language expresses the unconscious" (p. 30). "Complex metaphors are stories with many levels of meaning. Telling a story distracts the conscious mind and activates an unconscious search for meaning and resources" (p. 31). Jones believes that all clients communicate in metaphor. She explains that this form of language enables people to convey and cope with the depth of their feelings in a safe way.

Storytelling

In addition to telling stories to convey information to clients, therapists tell stories to establish rapport and to form personal connections. Specifically focusing on ordinary activities, stories allow clients to create a human connection to changes in the ordinary. The focus on the ordinary is the business of occupational therapy.

In addition to therapists' doing things for clients outside their formal role, Mattingly and Fleming (1994) found that therapists exchanged stories to promote an alliance and collaborative relationship with the client. They noted, "A similar strategy for creating personal bonds through exchange was evident in the exchange of stories of personal experience with clients. This was probably the most common strategy for building rapport, and most therapists were self-conscious and explicit with researchers about their use of personal stories in creating relationships with their clients" (p. 193). According to Mattingly and Fleming, therapists constantly reasoned about how much to reveal and make themselves the focus without losing the basic therapeutic structure where the therapist gives and the client receives treatment.

Images

Use of mental imagery is very common in occupational therapy. Images are used in a variety of ways, but two are most talked about: creating an image to visualize the person and using an image as a point of reference for recall. First, look at getting to know the person. Therapists talk a lot about having patients talk through their typical days to understand performance demands. Images of the patient are also found, as in finding clues to a person's life history, by scanning a patient's room. "When you go into a room, you form an image based on a few facts," says Debby Slater. Slater also comments, "You can't talk too much and you can't roll over them. You have to ask a few well-chosen questions and have a few responses on how you size up the situation. . . . Use of mental imagery, 'tell me about your day, what you do' is very effective. Then the person knows what occupational therapy is." Therapists also use images to link the patient's understanding of the problem to expected performance problems. The act of quickly formulating questions with a few cues and images in mind is truly an art. Mattingly (1998) astutely observes, "When a therapist asks the question, 'What story am I in?' she cannot sit back and wait for an answer. The question is posed in the midst of things at the same moment that action is required" (p. 160).

Second is the use of images as a point of reference. When therapy is working, an image is formed, the information is applied, and clients with children are able to refer to this in future similar situations. The image becomes a shorthand in the patient or parent's mind for a way to cope or adapt a situation. In working with mothers, Laura Snell believes the connection is made when parents come up with their own ideas. She gives two very good examples. "What can we do when the child is screaming in the park? How can he be calmed? He is a sensory kid, so what kinds of things will give him an outlet for those things? The mother may remember the 'chewies,' keeping the stroller moving—the therapist is thinking 'oral motor input, movement.'" According to Snell, "In this situation mom is very involved. I have spent time teaching so mother is thinking in a sensory framework. For example, she notices her child likes a tight cap on his head when he eats. She brings it up. She is an example of taking it and running with it."

TECHNIQUES

Five techniques characterize practice in all settings and with all populations: (1) selling, (2) giving back, (3) engaging the mood, (4) validating, and (5) holding. (See Information Checkpoint 3.3.) The therapist uses these techniques at various points in a session and over time. Although the processes and objectives may be similar, there is no stage-specific sequence for their use. Nevertheless, some techniques may be more appropriate to individuals and for problems natural to the beginning of the therapeutic relationship, while others are more often used at termination. The therapist must sense the need as well as make a judgement on a moment-to-moment and case-by-case basis.

Selling: Getting the Person to Buy In through Use of Mental Imagery and in Talking the Task

Therapists told me the client's understanding of occupational therapy was essential. It is as if the therapist is selling a service. The selling, or getting the person to buy in, is attempted with mental imagery and in talking the task. Therapists most often use these strategies during initial meetings when therapeutic goals and treatment plans are established. Mattingly (1998) concurs with my analysis when she says, "Much of therapy is directed, through actions more than words, to seducing clients to struggle with failing bodies" (p. 164).

First, the therapist explains the therapeutic activity in relation to therapeutic goals and at a level commensurate with the best of the patient's understanding. This involves connecting information from professionals and family members or other significant people with patients' reports of their own problems in functioning. For example, in the hospital, the therapist conveys to the patient the connection between medical information from the doctor and the patient's own concerns related to his or her functioning at home or work. In an outpatient, pediatric setting, the therapist may be selling occupational therapy to the parent. In that case, the therapist is giving information to the parent related to observations from a teacher, the therapist, child, other family member, or the parent him or herself. This requires the therapist to move between a person-specific (person-centered) approach and diagnostic-specific approach.

Talking about the connection has elements of both teaching and providing a reality orientation. To understand the impact of the illness or injury, both the therapist and the client, student, caretaker, teacher, or family member must envision the person, not just the ADL (activity of daily living). The therapist does this by exploring with the person the meaning of the problem or disability in terms of how it affects the person's daily life. This is often an unfamiliar process. As the person may have a cognitive impairment, be thinking in concrete ways, be confused, or be anxious, for example, the therapist uses mental imagery, according to Debby Slater, to take the person through the task, as Dalit Waller puts it. (See Critical Case Question 3.1.)

With imagery and task analysis, the therapist is helping the person to concretize the situation. In using imagery the therapist says, for example, "Imagine you are in your kitchen and reaching for the plates. How far up would you have to reach, and so on and so forth." When the parent or client begins to bring similar situations to the therapist, the process is considered successful. For example, in using task analysis, mom reports that her child is restless in his infant seat, yet she notices that he calms down when wearing his ski hat. In the next session, she happily reports that the family had a wonderful dinner when she put a hat on her son for the duration of the meal! The client, the teacher, or, in this case, the mother is successful when he or she learns about the condition and can independently conduct a task analysis and adapt the situation.

Chapter 3:   The Occupational Therapy Practice

Giving Back: Giving Back Control through Choice and Collaboration

Therapists talk a lot about collaboration. This client-centered approach is carefully orchestrated and not random. Collaborating with the client and giving choice is getting to know what clients are *really* like and what their goals are. Through the process of always giving the person choices, the therapist believes he or she is giving back control.

By empathizing in a particular manner, the therapist "gives back control." This form of empathy has an added dimension to that described by psychotherapists and reviewed earlier. In occupational therapy, empathy is perceived as giving choices and helping people to understand how these choices influence their function. The empathy comes through the process of giving choice in areas of function, and ultimately that is what gives back control. In occupational therapy, empathy involves an action, not emotional and intellectual understanding alone. This is a crucial difference from other definitions of empathy. As explained, the client comes to learn the meaning of the problem or disability through a revising of the mental image of self. The client, with the therapist's help, projects the future through imagining the lived or earlier occupational roles, activities, and ways of functioning. Through the exchange just described, the client comes to know the revised self-image or new self and has the opportunity for choice and control.

It appears paradoxical to believe one can give back control. Rather, is this an illusion of control? It is like saying I will give you freedom. How can one give something that cannot be given but is experienced? Is there control only when the person can act on his or her own will, or is the experience of perceiving choice sufficient? Although this may appear to be a purely philosophical question, it is central to the art of interactive reasoning in occupational therapy. The concerns are an outgrowth of the humanistic existential philosophical roots of the profession. It is through the therapist-client interaction that the therapist facilitates or enables the client to function through making choices. (See Critical Case Question 3.2.)

Engaging the Mood: Engaging the Person as Person through Mood in the Moment to Moment

Timing and *sensing* are terms often used when therapists are pushed to explain what they actively do to engage client, student, or family member. Therapists speak about responding to the "person as person" in the "moment to moment." In addition to time is the appropriate use of prompts. The sensing takes into account observing needs and then modifying the interactions and the environment through cues. It is a process of adapting the activity, interaction, environment, and sometimes equipment to match the person.

The process involves establishing rapport without lag time. According to Sue Brown, it is a quick judgement that takes into account knowledge of the person's behavioral status and cognitive capacity to comprehend and process information. The therapist is reflecting back the client's mood while trying to alter it to engage the person. As Laura Impemba, OTR/L, of Health South Braintree, explains, "I try to adapt myself and reflect back [the patients'] mood and at the same time I am trying to alter it to engage them." The therapist is always implicitly evaluating whether the interaction will stagnate or facilitate the patient's therapeutic advancement. A therapist's comment, paraphrased statement, or question, each seemingly an extemporaneous act, is carefully monitored for its effect. Thayer McCain, OTR/L, private practitioner of Thriving at Home, says, "I throw something out and see if it resonates." Although McCain makes this seem simple, the therapist must observe carefully and respond quickly. If the therapist is successful, the person will feel validated in the moment and is thereby engaged in a therapeutic process.

Validating: Validating through Clarifying

As just explained, engaging the person through mood in the moment is a means to establishing rapport. If successful, this strategy can be bridged with further validating the person through clarifying. Clarifying is active listening—reflecting back what you are hearing to see whether it is accurate.

The process of clarifying that you are not misunderstanding is in itself validating to the person. It is not that the therapist validates in direct ways. It is in the act of checking the understanding that the person feels understood and the importance of concern is agreed upon or sanctioned as real.

Holding: Providing a Holding Environment by Keeping the Personal Non–Therapy-Based Conversation Going

In occupational therapy, as found in the literature, and in these interviews, practitioners often tell stories about what they call the "ordinary." These stories may be about the therapist's own life or other events such as those reported in local, national or international news. "Through the non–therapy-based conversation, the therapist keeps the personal aspect going with the work," says Laura Impemba. The work involves activities for muscle strengthening and improving range of motion, balance, coordination, cognitive skills, and so forth. The therapist's aim is to provide a holding environment or supportive container for the patient. The conversation, or "holding," is believed, from what I was told, to help clients do the component work. Nevertheless, it in itself may be therapeutic. In Sharrott's (1983) words, the everyday activities and talk that constitute occupational therapy "play a significant role in the client's maintenance and legitimation of the newly reconstructed everyday world of reality" (p. 229).

It is not surprising that the "work" is pejoratively called the work because it refers to component work. Therapists and clients may enjoy the conversation and therefore not perceive it as work or therapy. Although the conversation may be equally therapeutic, it may not be viewed as a legitimate reimbursement service for occupational therapy. Nevertheless, the talk serves several therapeutic purposes and is not trivial or idle discussion.

Seasoned therapists observe that students and novice practitioners may experience difficulty knowing how to tell stories related to the ordinary without becoming friends with the client. In relating on a professional level, the therapist maintains a boundary that may be transparent to the beginner. A rule of thumb is to tell stories only if they will enhance the client's progress. Further, the therapist should ask whether this is a projection of my needs, a tonic for me, or in the service of the client's real or imagined needs. Finally, it is useful to analyze and validate the client's understanding of stories. Misunderstandings can occur as a result of cognitive impairments such as concrete thinking. Misinterpretations also occur because emotional states may lead to desires and fantasies that cannot be realistically fulfilled. Distortions in thinking can also result from feelings of depression and anxiety common in populations that occupational therapists encounter. (See Critical Case Question 3.3.)

In addition to storytelling, the therapist provides a holding environment or containment through feedback, redirecting, and cues. The therapist should first ask, What are the emotional needs of the person on a developmental continuum? For example, if the person appears very needy and is demanding, it would suggest he or she needs cues offering a caring response. However, the person may not be able to tolerate the attention. If the client is rejecting, does he or she fear closeness, or is he or she desperately seeking attention but fears asking or being dependent? Without appearing simplistic, it is useful to consider an approach avoidance equation. By analyzing the balance between the wish and the fear, the therapist can gauge what the client will tolerate and therefore the containment. The feedback comes in the form of what the therapist says and does or does not say or do. The person is redirected by the therapist's fulfillment of the emotional need of the moment. For example, when the client says "Go away, I hate you," does he or she mean "Please stay, but I fear I love you" or "I truly want you to disappear"? More than likely, in such a case, the client would run if you were too interested and caring. To contain, the therapist must tentatively offer to stay or return at another time. By waiting and observing in silence the client has an opportunity to take as much as he or she can tolerate.

ETHICAL DILEMMAS

It is expected that management issues, such as the need to document a treatment plan for reimbursement, will to some degree force the use of particular techniques. This problem is expected to grow as third-party payers increase control over the management of service delivery and put monetary gain over quality of care. The ethics involved in shaping the treatment process for the purpose of reimbursement requires careful attention and therapist examination. The therapist must ask several questions: Is this in the client's best interests? Is the expectation realistic based on past experience and research? Is the process being dictated by the client's needs or the therapist's own psychological or social circumstances? (See Information Checkpoint 3.4.)

BACK TO MRS. SMITH

To engage Mrs. Smith in occupational therapy, the practitioner first needed to understand what was important to her client. By conveying acceptance, the therapist was able to build a trusting relationship with her client. Over time, Mrs. Smith learned how to take care of herself and promote her own health. She resumed her family caretaker role and at the same time stopped smoking, joined a support group for people with chronic respiratory diseases, and used the energy conservation techniques to enable her maximum level of activity.

SUMMARY

Occupational therapists' unique perspective on interactive reasoning was presented. Five themes and five techniques were identified and discussed. The themes included the following: (1) active participation and collaboration, (2) engaging/connecting with the person and creating a holding environment, (3) exploring and interpreting motives as well as occupation-based meanings, (4) listening, and (5) understanding and use of narrative/symbolic. Five techniques characterized practice in all settings and with all populations: (1) selling, (2) giving back, (3) engaging the mood, (4) validating, and (5) holding. The themes and techniques of interactive reasoning will be applied in the remaining chapters. (See Information Checkpoint 3.5.)

REFLECTIVE QUESTIONS

- Describe themes related to occupational therapists' concerns about interactive reasoning. Reflect upon occupational therapists' experience and imagine yourself in the situation. How would you feel? What concerns would you have as a practitioner?
- Identify techniques employed by occupational therapists in interacting with their clients, students, and families. Imagine receiving this care. How would you feel? What concerns might you have?
- How do pressures around reimbursement for services affect therapists? What are their ethical concerns? Reflect upon your own ethics. How would you manage should conflict arise between your own beliefs and expectations of others?
- In addition to employing their own philosophy and methodologies, occupational therapists have borrowed and integrated ideas from related fields. Which assumptions seem similar to you? How would you characterize differences between the occupational therapist's perspective and that of individuals in other fields? Reflecting upon your own experience in receiving health care, describe the methodologies you imagine were used and your relative degree of satisfaction.

INFORMATION CHECKPOINTS

3.1. TYPES OF HELPING

Norrby and Bellner (1995) conducted a study in Sweden similar to my research for this book. They interviewed therapists to find out perceptions of their therapeutic encounters with patients. Three types of helping portrayed therapists' concerns:

1. Basic professional-oriented helping (create professional help)
   - Self-knowledge
   - Empathy
   - Life and professional experience

2. Understanding-oriented helping (understand the patient)
   - Communication
   - Safety
   - Respect
3. Action-oriented helping (activate the client)
   - Motivating
   - Strengthening of self
   - Adapting to the individual reality

3.2. INTERVIEW-GENERATED THEMES RELATED TO INTERACTIVE REASONING

ACTIVE PARTICIPATION AND COLLABORATION

- Offering control by creating choices
- Client-centered
- Role of occupational therapy
- Client insight into impact on function
- Joint problem solving

ENGAGING/CONNECTING WITH THE PERSON AND CREATING A HOLDING ENVIRONMENT

- Trust
- Hope
- Empathy
- Mutual regard

EXPLORING AND INTERPRETING MOTIVES AS WELL AS OCCUPATION-BASED MEANINGS

- The individual
- The individual and the group as a whole

LISTENING

- Active listening (cue identification)
- Validating and genuineness
- Affirmation of the client
- Empathic connection and rapport
- Goal setting
- Moment to moment

UNDERSTANDING AND USE OF NARRATIVE/SYMBOLIC

- Life history
- Metaphors
- Storytelling
- Images

3.3. FIVE TECHNIQUES CHARACTERISTIC OF PRACTICE

1. Selling: Getting the person to buy in through use of mental imagery and talking the task
2. Giving back: Giving back control through choice and collaboration
3. Engaging the mood: Engaging the person as person through mood in the moment to moment
4. Validating: Validating through clarifying
5. Holding: Providing a holding environment by keeping the personal non–therapy-based conversation going

3.4. ETHICAL ISSUES

Ethical issues arise during the course of the therapeutic interview. The therapist must select a course that is in the client's best interests. See AOTA (1999) "Standards of Practice" and "Guide to Occupational Therapy Practice" for more detail.

3.5. THEMES AND TECHNIQUES OF INTERACTIVE REASONING

FIVE INTERVIEW-GENERATED THEMES ON OCCUPATIONAL THERAPY INTERACTIVE REASONING

- Active participation and collaboration
- Engaging/connecting with the person and creating a holding environment
- Exploring and interpreting motives as well as occupation-based meanings
- Listening
- Understanding and use of narrative/symbolic

FIVE TECHNIQUES CHARACTERISTIC OF OCCUPATIONAL THERAPY PRACTICE

- Selling: Getting the person to buy in through use of mental imagery and talking the task
- Giving back: Giving back control through choice and collaboration
- Engaging the mood: Engaging the person as person through mood in the moment to moment
- Validating: Validating through clarifying
- Holding: Providing a holding environment by keeping the personal non–therapy-based conversation going

CRITICAL CASE QUESTIONS

3.1. Should the therapist mention the smell of cigarettes directly to Mrs. Smith or her family? Would it be better to describe a scenario to Mrs. Smith where she is smoking and unable to care for her grandchildren? How would you help this client understand the effect of her medical problem on her future functioning?

3.2 Mrs. Smith's cognitive functioning appears changed since she was hospitalized. This may be due to anoxia or the effects of living in a hospital. Mrs. Smith reports to understand that when doing housework, to conserve energy, she will need to do a little at a time and set priorities for what she hopes to accomplish during the day. When she returned home, there was no change from her earlier daily routine. Is Mrs. Smith in control? How would you intervene, and why?

3.3. When Mrs. Smith was in the hospital as an inpatient, the occupational therapist found Mrs. Smith sulking at her bedside. Confused by her change in behavior from previous encounters, the therapist recalled a story she told her client yesterday. The story was about how, in order to save time, unlike her mother who is an excellent cook, the therapist makes chicken soup from bouillon cubes. What might you speculate about Mrs. Smith's reaction? How would you intervene in this situation? Would you start with the assumption that her response is in reaction to the story or draw different hypotheses? What would they be? At the time, the therapist was trying to reassure the client that there were ways to conserve energy and still cook.

KEY TERMS

CONDITIONAL REASONING

"Conditional reasoning is used to revise treatment moment to moment to meet the clients' needs. This revision is done with an eye to the clients' current and possible future contexts" (Neistadt, 1998, p. 228).

INTERACTIVE REASONING

According to Neistadt (1998), "interactive reasoning yields an understanding of what the disease or disability means to the client (i.e., the client's illness experience). Interactive reasoning also encompasses the interpersonal interactions between therapists and clients" (p. 229). In their study of modes of reasoning, Fleming and Mattingly (1994) found that "interactive reasoning is used to help the therapist to interact with and better understand the person. Interactive reasoning takes place during face-to-face encounters between the therapist and client. It is the form of reasoning that therapists employ when they want to better understand the client as a person. There are many reasons why a therapist might want to know the person better. The therapist might want to know how the person feels about the treatment at the moment; or what the client is like as a person, either out of sheer interest or in order to more finely tailor the treatment to his or her specific needs or preferences. Further, the therapist may be interested in this person, in order to better understand the experience of the disability from the person's own point of view" (p. 17).

NARRATIVE REASONING

"Narrative reasoning yields the client's occupational history (i.e., his or her life history as told through preferred activities, habits, and roles). Narrative reasoning also encompasses the client and therapist's shared story (i.e., how the therapist and client will incorporate the client's activity preferences into intervention to build a meaningful future for the client)" (Neistadt, 1998, pp. 227–228).

PRAGMATIC REASONING

"Pragmatic reasoning is used to consider all of the practical issues that affect occupational therapy services: the treatment environment; the therapist's values, knowledge, abilities, and experiences; the client's social and financial resources; and the client's potential discharge environments. Therapists use this type of reasoning to decide what is possible to do for a particular client in a given treatment setting" (Neistadt, 1998, p. 228).

PROCEDURAL REASONING

"Procedural reasoning is the process of defining clients' diagnostically related occupational performance area, performance component, and performance context problems and selecting appropriate interventions" (Neistadt, 1998, p. 228).

THE PRACTICE ENVIRONMENTS

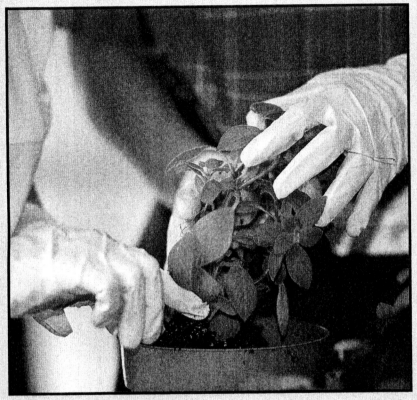

The Power Alliance: An Interactive Reasoning Approach to the Practitioner-Client Relationship

*P*art II takes the reader to the settings in which occupational therapists practice. It includes three chapters that describe very different ecological and socioeconomic perspectives. In chapter 4, institutional environments of the inpatient unit and outpatient service provide a context for interactions embedded in a medical model. Although the occupational therapist's role in the acute care setting is diminishing, the hospital remains a fundamental element in health care service delivery. In chapter 5, the school and educational settings become the context from which interactive practice is presented. Because of legislation in the United States, large proportions of occupational

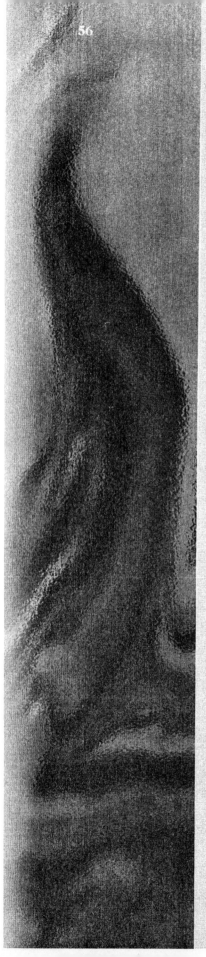

therapists are now working with children in the schools. Chapter 6 concludes Part II by taking the reader to community settings.

It is the vision of many occupational therapists that the future of practice will evolve in community settings. For a variety of reasons, both economic and demographic, the practitioner is now working with clients in nonmedical settings such as the home and office. As these new environments emerge and are developed, the occupational therapist is increasingly acting as a consultant. Thus, the interactive process is not with the client alone but with the client and a teacher, the board, or a community agency. In recognizing these systematic differences, the clinical reasoning of the occupational therapist is approached from the perspective of the individual, the institution, and the community.

INPATIENT AND OUTPATIENT HOSPITAL

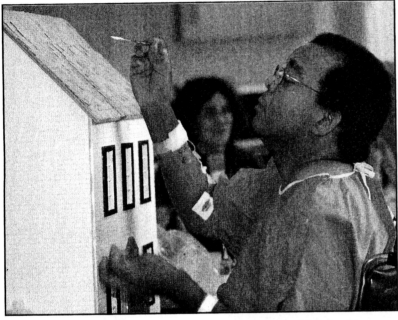

FIGURE 4.1   Giving Back Control through Occupation-Based Relationships

IDENTITY
By Alice Adelman Lowenstein
(copyright 2000, all rights reserved)

CASE STUDY
4.1

*T*his is a segment of Alice's story sent via e-mail February 13, 2000. Alice later requested that I mention that since she is healing, what I quoted won't be true for the rest of her life. She believes this was the way she felt for fourteen and a half years before she saw Joe Burstein, the acupuncturist who knows how to treat head-injured people (personal communication, Alice Lowenstein, May 4, 2000, electronic mail).

"... What I did do or didn't do wasn't my identity. My roles weren't my identity. How I cleaned up the house or didn't, or how I had parties or didn't, wasn't my identity. It was my style. The blessing of the accident is that I discovered the difference between style and identity. I discovered I was in a

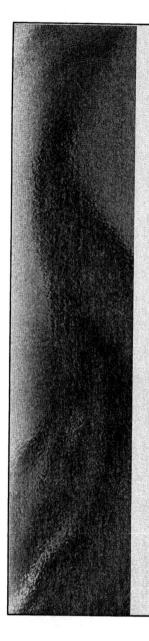

long process of learning how to take care of myself. Otherwise, my body wouldn't function and I couldn't do anything in any style but lay *[sic]* down on the bed and rest. . . .

Except sometimes even now, I get proud of how much I can do in a day, proud of all the impossible things I can do. After a few of those kinds of days, I have real trouble quieting down and relaxing. If I don't quiet down, then my body stops functioning. Maybe I get incontinent. My brain cannot remember to help me not shame myself. I just have to think about the bathroom, no coughing, just think and I'm going. Even if I try to willfully control myself I can't. . . .

Whether I liked it or not, after the accident I couldn't do things the old way. Still, the old patterns of thinking remained. The whole way of not knowing what a person is; what a person can reasonably expect of him or herself; how to be satisfied with doing a moderate amount of work for something; being satisfied with moderation and balance; all of this was simply what I didn't know.

I could not discover what a person was because of the confusion I had from my parents. They said they were parents. They said they were putting my needs first. They said they were doing things for me, but if I asked my mother for help, I then had to reassure her that she was a good mother because having a child asking for help meant she wasn't. I had to be in terrific need to begin asking my mother.

No matter what I did [it] was never good enough. I was never perfect. I thought as a child that if I were perfect, they would behave as loving, compassionate parents. My friend had parents who were similar to mine— loving excess, not knowing what is enough, not being in balance, not knowing how to take care of themselves, always asking the children to take care of them, to make them feel loved and important.

With all this old confusion I had the accident. Now I was a head-injured person. What is that? Is that a kind of person, like a just person, or a mensch? I was in a similar situation with my caregivers as I had been with my parents. They were getting money from the hospital, or from the insurance company; they were professionals with professional language and professional respect. They did know how to keep me alive. For that I am deeply grateful. . . ."

OVERVIEW

*T*his chapter includes examples from inpatient rehabilitation units and out-patient services in large community city and suburban acute care hospitals, locked inpatient psychiatric units and partial hospitalization programs in urban and suburban acute care hospitals, subacute and long-term care rehabilitation hospitals, and skilled nursing facilities (transitional care units). These examples involve situations where the occupational therapist works as a generic rehabilitation therapist and in discipline-specific roles. The process of interactive reasoning is portrayed in two broad types of service settings: the "traditional" inpatient unit where the therapist is working within a medical model and the outpatient setting where the client is living in the community.

Inpatient and outpatient hospital settings present unique dilemmas in working with clients. The effects of the medical model and institutional environment affect both the client and the therapist. Practice context has been found to influence occupational therapists' clinical reasoning in terms of type of activity intervention selected (Schell & Cervero, 1995). An analysis of the literature also indicates how those personal and practice context issues, such as therapists' skills, reimbursement, and availability of equipment, affect clinical reasoning and practice (Schell & Cervero, 1993).

As one can see in the chapter opening case study, because of the severity of medical situations, clients in hospitals and outpatient clinics may experience feeling grateful for being kept alive. Occupational therapists are in a role to encourage and instill hope in their clients. However, three problematic areas deserve careful attention: (1) depersonalization and loss of personal meaning, (2) distancing and diminishing clients, and (3) withholding information, consciously or by not knowing, and misuse of power (Peloquin, 1993). The former types of mistreatment are of particular concern in institutional environments that may in several ways foster this behavior in therapists. The environment and therapists' experiences and clinical reasoning strategies are presented in pages that follow. (See Critical Case Question 4.1.)

THE MEDICAL MODEL AND INSTITUTIONAL ENVIRONMENT

Inpatient and outpatient settings are for the most part driven by the medical model of service delivery. The person seeking help comes with symptoms and a perceived illness to be treated. The eradication of disease sets the metaphor for the patient-doctor relationship. The therapist becomes ancillary to a process of diagnosis and treatment or intervention around acute needs. The medical referral for occupational therapy services in the institutional environment is the initial link or connection to the patient. Those requiring compensatory or skills training because of a disability are eventually referred elsewhere for these occupational therapy services. It is only then that the occupational therapy client-clinician relationship is truly established.

DISPARITY OF POWER

In such an environment where there are experts and dependents—the clients—a hierarchical relationship is established. We see the symbolic nature of hospital and caregiver as authority, or parental, figure in the chapter opening case study. As Alice Lowenstein (2000) puts it, "I was in a similar situation with my caregivers as I had been with my parents." The client's "identity" and experience as a dependent is brought to the relationship with the "professionals." (See Critical Case Question 4.2.) The age of the client, cultural orientation, and type of condition are also reflected in the pattern of asking for and receiving care. We will see the particular relevance of age or, rather, developmental issues, in Part III, which discusses various populations.

Along with the client's transference response to the medical setting is the therapist's countertransference reaction. The therapeutic relationship is a dynamic process. A therapist's response to being in the authority role and the degree of comfort with this perceived or real power will vary. Rather than shared power, there is a danger in the therapist's being overly controlling with a client and family.

One can see from the case study that the symbolic meanings of roles as parent and child influence adult occupational behavior and attitudes in the client role. As a child, as Alice Lowenstein (2000) describes it, she was confused about her identity. Although her parents said they were putting her needs first, rather than express a need, Alice believed she had to first reassure her mother that she was a good mother. As a client, Alice was dependent upon the professionals and deeply grateful for being kept alive, yet in the situation, she was not sure what to reasonably expect in giving voice to her own needs or her identity. The institutional setting and client role in the hospital and clinic challenge the delicate psychological balance of prior adaptations. The outcome may be positive or negative. (See Critical Case Question 4.3.)

LAWS, POLICIES, RIGHTS OF CONSENT AND DISCLOSURE, CONTRACTS

The client's vulnerability in the institutional setting is due to a variety of factors. The disparity of power between the client and caregiver as well as between the individual and the institution is one concern. Therapists are advised to know the laws and policies governing their work and institution. Clients' rights to consent and disclosure are aimed at limiting their exposure to harm. The use of verbal and written contracts or agreements may be preliminary to interaction. Therapists report how they use hospital protocols in their introductory remarks with a client and in eliciting collaboration. The client has a right to know the aim and method of intervention. This requires the occupational therapist to explain and explore the process so that it has meaning to the client and significant others.

CHALLENGES OF THE INSTITUTIONAL ENVIRONMENT: SEXUALITY, BOUNDARIES AND CLOSENESS, DEATH AND DYING

For some practitioners, engaging the client in a collaborative process will be threatening, particularly if the client is very ill and medically dependent. For others, the ability to collaborate under such a circumstance will be more natural. Through clinical reasoning, the therapist uses internal and external cues from the client to discern patterns of need as well as means of responding.

As we will see in the therapists' reports, techniques take on a special meaning in the institutional environment. Working in a hospital, for example, the therapist interacts with the client at bedside. The client may feel sexually and emotionally exposed. As one sees in the opening case, the person may be concerned about losing control of body functions. The therapist needs to respect the person's vulnerability and the potential for feeling shame. Clear boundaries, respect for needs for closeness and distance, are particularly important in the institutional setting.

In this setting, the therapist may also regularly be exposed to the dying client and family members. Communicating with the dying and their families is an especially challenging situation (Purtilo & Haddad, 1996). Active listening is crucial, as one can expect fear and denial (Davis, 1998). The need to translate the person's concern into a meaningful plan of intervention requires acceptance, creativity, and skill.

TRANSLATING MEANING

As discussed in chapter 3, one of the major tasks for occupational therapists working in hospital settings is translating the meaning of the client's condition to the everyday world. Mattingly (1998) describes the challenge:

> Occupational therapy is a "ritual of the everyday" played out in the clinical world, the world of the not everyday. . . . Therapists often translate the esoteric language of medicine to the ordinary language of common sense in helping patients understand their condition. This insistence on the ordinary and the "normal" carries the symbolic message that people are capable of making the transition from patient to member of society, assuming in some fashion the roles and cares and community that characterize life without disability. (pp. 165–166)

THE EXPERIENCED THERAPIST AND THE NOVICE

Experienced therapists use knowledge gained from previous situations to make sense of the situations before them. This clinical task is more difficult for the novice. Robertson (1999) calls this process "pattern matching" (p. 22). She also observes that experts use "clustering" and "cue and pattern recognition" to help frame a clinical problem. It is from this framework, according to Robertson (1999), that boundaries can be set and decisions made. (See Information Checkpoint 4.1.) (See Critical Case Question 4.4.)

According to Fleming (1994), "Experienced OTs seem to have the uncommon ability to treat the physical condition objectively while simultaneously understanding the person's subjective experience of his or her condition" (p. 125). Fleming believes that the integration of the interactive and procedural aspects had more to do with values and role perception than experience or amount of time on the job. She also explains that conditional reasoning involves the therapist's thinking about the whole condition (person, illness, and meaning of the illness in context of person, family, physical, and social realms), how the condition could change (proposed, revised condition), and the imagined state—that which is conditional upon the client's participation. Fleming further notes that this type of reasoning guides the phenomenological aspects of practice and is more often found in experienced therapists. "We postulate that in using conditional reasoning, the therapist reflects upon the success or failure of the clinical encounter from both the procedural and interactive standpoints and attempts to integrate the two" (p. 133). Occupational therapists who were interviewed identified many strategies they used in interacting with clients in the inpatient or outpatient setting, including overturning preconceived notions, engaging the client, instilling hope, employing creativity wisely, facilitating success, interviewing effectively, being prepared, and looking inward.

ACTIVE PARTICIPATION AND COLLABORATION

Client-centered therapy requires active participation of the client in the process of evaluation and intervention. In occupational therapy, a collaborative relationship is sought from the beginning. It is not unusual, however, to find that the client or family members are resistant to collaboration. This is especially true in acute care hospital settings where the clients are very ill. Clients may feel frightened, unable to perceive the value of occupational therapy, be focused on basic survival needs such as breathing, be disoriented, and so on. The therapist's primary challenge is in building a therapeutic alliance from the first contact and onward.

The best interactive practice occurs when collaboration and trust exist between therapist and client. "When I think of a good collaboration," says Regina Doherty, OTR/L, of the Massachusetts General Hospital, "the therapist asks the patient what is important for him or her, and the patient can identify certain goals he or she would like to work on. It is a team effort." As Deborah Slater, OTR/L, of the New England Baptist Hospital, straightforwardly explains, "Occupational therapy is very collaborative. You have to have the person buy in."

The best therapists are thoughtful about their approach to the client and periodically review their techniques. "Our staff has been revisiting the client-centered approach, starting with the therapeutic relationship," says Jim Sellers, OTR/L, of the New England Sinai Hospital and Rehabilitation Center. "I am currently working with 'resource clinicians' to look at our evaluation tool, which is very component-driven and uses lots of checklists. Some people use the checklist and get information they may not necessarily need because it is on the form. That sort of pre-fab approach is what we are looking to go beyond. People

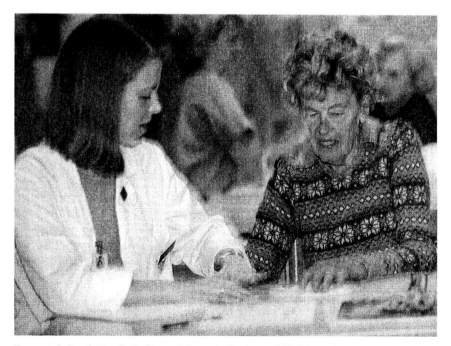

FIGURE 4.2 Giving Back Control through Choice and Collaboration

don't really trust it. <u>You must start with what has meaning to the person.</u> The rest—range of motion, endurance, etc.—will follow. Finding out what the patient needs the most works best in an outpatient clinic, because people who go back home really need to have a sense of control. In working with burn patients, it took everything I had to tell them I must do this and it is going to hurt, but I have to do it. I always try to think about the elements of choice and control, especially in a hospital, where there is little of either."

OVERTURNING PRECONCEIVED NOTIONS

"If there is a place in hell for those who supported component land, I will have to spend some time there," admits Sellers. "I really pushed for it earlier. I pushed for physical agent modalities. Now I wouldn't. In acute care, I thought you had to 'fix' things. Now I am very embarrassed. I was worried I was asleep in class when they taught me how to fix things. One patient I treated had a stroke, and although I tried my best, I could not help him regain his function. He thought I didn't like him! Then it came to me—there is me, and I have worked hard [as therapist], and there is you, and you have worked hard [as patient], and there is Mother Nature, and we can capitalize on what Mother Nature has given us to work with. If I had been 'with' him rather than 'on' him in terms of my approach, then I believe therapy would have evolved in a more realistic and timely way. It would have been a collaboration. The expectation of myself as a therapist, my insecurities, and my naivete at the time did not allow me to trust myself.

"[Therapists need] to clear their mind before they talk to the person," says Sellers. "It reminds me of when I was in art school: Approaching a patient is similar to the way the artist focuses on the blank canvas. Before you say anything to the person is like facing the canvas before you decide where the first stroke goes."

Jim Sellers's coworkers at New England Sinai Hospital and Rehabilitation Center also express a need to go beyond the set protocol. "We will not actively address a goal unless there is active participation with the patient," says coworker Jennifer Saylor, OTR/L. "I have done this [person-centered approach] in an interview. We used to tell the patient, 'This is what OT is at Sinai.' There used to be standard questions, such as: 'Do you drive?' It was almost a speech. Now I ask, 'What is important to you? Tell me what you want to do.' I can tell in the first few moments if I will need to 'lead' rather than 'follow.' Usually the patient has the approach, 'You need to treat me!' In that case, I try to switch it around to involve the patient."

ENGAGING THE CLIENT

Sinai coworker Julie Taberman, OTR/L, says, "The best interactive reasoning occurs when patients are really engaged with the activity. They are really enjoying the activity and they are stretching themselves. It is often not what they have done before. It may be something that is a little bit of a challenge, and they are growing. Today, for example, I was working with someone with COPD [chronic obstructive pulmonary disease] who couldn't stay on her feet. I was trying to get her to stand while distracting her. So we were playing field hockey, which she used to play, and she managed to stay on her feet for two minutes. She was having fun. She had been thinking about what was important to her and not her breath. She was taking a lot of breaks. She was pacing herself. I was trying to reinforce what was happening. Things were perking along."

Fellow coworker Michael Davison, OTR/L, says, "I still like to follow MOHO [model of human occupation] in terms of roles. I generally stay away from the biomechanical-adaptation model. When I first started to practice, I leaned toward the biomechanical. You have the diagnostic-specific approach versus the person-specific approach. I prefer starting with the latter and focus on what is really important to the person who has a shorter length of stay. I like the COPM [Canadian Occupational Performance Measure], as it is motivating in its focus on what is important to the individual. Teaching and reality orientation are used to help motivate the person. This is rapport-building. 'I really can't help you with this, I can help you with that. It appears you are really not ready to . . . and I would like to come back in a few days when you are ready and it is convenient for you.' So much is giving back control. I always break it down to say, 'This is what I can help you with and I am more concerned with . . . for when you go home you will have to. . . .' Client-centered and human occupation are the key approaches I use. This involves gathering insight into the problem, questioning people, providing an explanation of what we do, asking if they know if someone else has the problem and how it affects them. It is being client-centered at its best."

Yet another Sinai coworker, Linda McGettigan, OTR/L, also advocates using the client-centered approach, which involves asking, "What are the patient's values?" McGettigan says, "It is hard to describe because it really is moment to moment. I may not go through with a plan because the patient may be overwhelmed. Here we do not have to practice around scores. Instead, our emphasis is on adjusting our responses to engage people in some goal that is important in their daily functioning. It is responding to the person as a person. A COTA I know says it well: 'I want to treat the person like my grandparent, and respect the person, giving the person time to talk and not talking when he or she is talking.' You get better information when time is allowed. And it really isn't that much more time."

INSTILLING HOPE

Janet Kahane, OTR/L, of Newton Wellesley Hospital, finds that the best interactive practice happens when the relationship with the client is going well and there is a sense that there is something the therapist can provide the client with. "There is the feeling that I am there to help the patient, a sense of helpfulness and hopefulness, something that the patient can buy into and wants to work on. Patients make suggestions, and I help them accomplish their goals. We identify what patients want to accomplish by the time they leave the hospital."

At the start of therapy, Kahane introduces herself and explains how she is part of the treatment team. She also describes the purpose of occupational therapy in relation to what brought the client in to the hospital. "There may be a resistance, a guardedness with psychiatric patients," she continues. "They need to have a clear understanding of what we are offering them. The therapist needs to instill a feeling of hopefulness before patients can start to feel better about an area they may have neglected. We give them a questionnaire ahead of time. This sets the tone. The questions focus on their performance of ADL tasks, goals, and coping skills. I also say I want to go over the schedule of activities on the unit. My theory is we need to get them in the door so they can see what others are doing. It gives them a sense of control, of its being their choice, and they understand the expectations. They say that is helpful."

In many hospital settings, occupational therapists function under physician orders and get referrals to the occupational therapy setting. "We are really consultants," says Pat Keck, OTR/L, of the Beth Israel Deaconess Medical Center in Boston. "The key to effective interactive therapy is in the first few moments: showing dignity and respect and focusing on what is important to the patient. For example, we might say, 'Your surgeon referred you to me, this is what occupational therapy is, and this is what the others on the team do.' A lot of time is spent educating the patient about the role of occupational therapy. We explain how it relates to his or her reason for being in the hospital. This approach gives the patient a sense of having control and autonomy. We use the COPM in the initial interview because it goes to that element very quickly. I think in the best interactive practice, the patient is an equal and participates in a dialogue."

USING TEAM EFFECTIVELY

The best interactive practice takes place through the treatment team, maintains Liz Freeman, OTR/L, also with Beth Israel Deaconess Medical Center. "I see things going well in my mind when the patient is the coach. The patient is empowered to guide his or her treatment. We are facilitators of their objectives. There are so many times when patients are surrounded by six experts. They look so small. In a group, teaching, and learning activities, is when they are proactive."

Several things go on simultaneously in the best interactive practice, say occupational therapists. "[Clients] give me information about such things as pain and how their program is working," says Carol (Harmon) Mahoney, OTR/L, of the Massachusetts General Hospital. "They feel like they can tell me if they need a change. There is an honesty and directness on the patient's part. There is a sense of humor. It is as though we have made a good deal together. I agree to do this, and they are willing to do that. We are willing to do this together. I spend a lot of time on patient education, what to expect, and how the systems at the hospital work."

ENGAGING/CONNECTING AND CREATING A HOLDING ENVIRONMENT

Occupational therapists emphasize acceptance as key to engaging with a client. They look to the person's identity to understand what is required to promote feelings of safety and involvement. This requires flexibility on the part of the therapist, as shifts in mood and occupational interests can be expected during the course of a hospitalization or outpatient treatment.

Many occupational therapists say they use their psychosocial training in the acute care setting. "The therapist gears the explanation of occupational therapy to the patient's personality," says Regina Doherty. "The patient feels like giving feedback to the therapist. The experienced therapist knows when to push the patient, as compared with the novice therapist, who might want to bring something up right away."

Therapists say they can sense when they are successful in their approach, but they do not stop working at making the session work. "There is contentment with the situation, [although] there never really is contentment," says Mike Miller, OTR/L, with Spaulding Rehabilitation Hospital. "You are really on guard because of the possibility of changes in a patient's medical condition or other life situations. If that happens, we have to set new goals. There is always the possibility of change. When it is working and everything is ideal, then there definitely is a flow and there definitely is a sense of satisfaction. You feel you are connecting with the person."

Occupational therapists say using such concepts as giving a client a sense of control and choice and building a sense of mutual trust and respect, which they borrow from such theorists as Maslow, helps them apply interactive reasoning. "You do have to give people control, but it is difficult to establish trust," says Jim Sellers. "And you have to learn to accept the variety of people and sizes and backgrounds. Having a healthy respect for differences is really important. It shows that you have some cultural competence and some cultural sensitivity; that is really important. If you start here, the rest will fall into place. You have to be open enough to finding this exciting, interesting, and fun. You have to be intimate. This is far away from 'I'm OK, you're OK.'"

EMPLOYING CREATIVITY WISELY

The long-term client needs special consideration. "My classic advice is you ultimately have to be creative with long-term patients," says Jennifer Saylor. "So I have really taken a more leisure time approach and given more emphasis to the quality of life. It is more patient-driven, around how the person can improve the quality of their [sic] life. When I started to feel hopeless about the patient's care in reaction to a person's feeling that way, then I realized I had to be creative in the things she chose. There was a lot of gradation involved. I had her direct more of the team by having her tell them what she needed. This was a real revelation for the staff. She was perceived as less needy. She felt that she was more in control. When the patient directed what she needed, the nursing staff had to spend less time with her. The nursing staff was shocked that this worked. The patient, now discharged, is still following this approach."

The basic occupational therapy skill of analyzing an activity or task helps many therapists break down what needs to be done in therapy. "A lot of it is task analysis," says Julie Taberman. "What will they need to do when they go home? What level of care will be needed? What things can we work on now, and what things won't we be able to change? What can we adapt, and what can we compensate for? A lot of the answers are available from the family. It is problem solving. The process has to be fluid. Things are not immediately obvious when you start working with a person. The goals may have to be amended, depending upon what the patient says he or she wants. As much as we learned clinical reasoning at school, nothing prepares you for it. On-the-job experience is what it is. I don't think you can short-cut that. You need the experience of juggling what the patient needs with what the family is saying and with setting goals. I think a lot of it changes as you work with the patient. It is a tacit process, and it is not formal."

Anticipating what the client will need at home and trying to meet the client by working in the clinic are two different things, say therapists. "I am looking for connecting the goals to what we are doing here," says Linda McGettigan. "One [woman], for example, had a humeral fracture, and she was having great difficulty accepting it. She said, 'All I did was cooking and cleaning.' So one day I brought in a deck of cards, and she said, 'Wow, this is what I did when I waited for my husband.' Then we used the cards, and she had to hold them and was involved in the treatment. It comes down to looking for a connection to what motivates people; sometimes it requires looking for what they are not saying. When they say, 'No one ever asked me what was important to me,' is when you know your approach is working."

Much of interactive reasoning is intuitive, say therapists. "I know a lot from the patients' facial reactions," continues McGettigan. "I don't think that any of the theories are really going to help, like NDT, unless we look at patients and what is going on with them first."

USING LIFE EXPERIENCES

Some therapists borrow from other aspects of their lives to make their interactions more effective. "The experience of parenting is my model," says Janet Kahane. "If people cannot make decisions, you tell them what to do. It is not always collaborative. It requires taking control when they are unclear or confused, being more directive, as you would with a child. Whether it is in a group or one to one, you make it a safe environment. It is the sense that the patients are here to get help in the setting, and this is what they have to do. I want to engage them at whatever level they are, first of all to get them in the door, by not being overbearing, and to start to develop the therapeutic relationship. I use a smile. It sounds manipulative, but it's not. I think being warm and engaging is a help. I might say, 'I know this is not where you want to be.' A big part of it is in acknowledging, validating, and understanding where they are."

"My philosophy is to be a patient advocate," says Carol Mahoney. "I try to listen to the patient and understand cultural differences, to work out goals and give the patient more responsibility. By looking at their body language, their eyes, I ask if they are on pain medications, what their expressions are conveying, how comfortable they are. If someone was in a lot of pain, for example, I would explain a lot more before using therapeutic touch. They are in need of more control. I might spend more time explaining things to the family. I might demonstrate what I would do, using the patient's non-affected side. This allows the person to gain trust. I also would explain things so that the patient wants to tell me what is going on, so that they have more control."

Some people interviewed say their experience as therapists allows them to become almost automatic in their response. "I might prescribe pacing," says Liz Freeman. "If someone was looking agitated and restless, I would think about safety. I would not want the person to emotionally explode in a group. I look to what is natural and can be done in a face-saving way. I think some of it has to do with safety and educating patients about coping techniques. We are always trying to improve the patient's insight into stress triggers. It involves analyzing and adapting the activity and teaching the person how to respond."

FACILITATING SUCCESS

"Often I try to engage the person by helping me," continues Freeman. "His or her role becomes one of assisting me. It is ultimately that I want the experience to be successful because that is going to be motivating. If therapy works, it should make the patient feel successful, valued, included, and it should ultimately result in reduced stress. The most therapeutic thing is when, for example, patients order a pizza on their own. They collect the money, do the calling and the serving. The natural activity is so much more meaningful. Patients are using their strengths; they are in control. Another time, the patients decided to order Chinese food and gave the task to a man. He came to me and said, 'I can't do this.' He was overwhelmed even at the thought of figuring out how to take the orders and collect the money. He needed help breaking down the task, asking for help, and so forth. That was where I could help. I think flow is when we are doing something and not just talking about it. In a one-on-one, I become a facilitator, when there is some sort of activity that feels the best. 'Let's not just talk about volunteering, let's get on the phone and set it up.'"

While experienced therapists have access to a variety of tools with which to approach therapy, effectiveness in interactive practice often comes down to the personal relationship, they say. "From my experience, the best interactive practice is when you make a connection with the patient," says Dan Kerls, OTR/L, Newton Wellesley Hospital. "I ask the patients, especially the older ones, what they do during the day. They may say they have a hobby. I try to relate to some part of their life. It makes them trust more. From what I have seen, patients often give the therapist a hard time at first. I use humor. They laugh back. Then they ask more about my life and others I have treated. They ask if I know anyone who has had their problem, such as 'Have you ever treated anyone with this? Did they go back to work?' Sometimes they want to be your friend, and it is difficult to set boundaries. I tend to use a lot of reality testing rather than browbeating them with medical facts. With the resistant people, I reiterate their own goals and ask, 'How will you do that with this condition?' I try to empower them, have them problem-solve."

When the interactive process is at its best, therapists can sense that something very effective is happening. "You can always tell best interactive practice by the conversation between the patient and therapist," says Deborah Slater. "They really are in sync. You know it when you see it, the therapist who is really effective. When you have a successful interaction, it is as if you are telling the patient, 'You and I are in this together.' There is a dialogue. This may or may not work, but if not, we will just have to readjust."

OFFERING CHOICES

Some therapists emphasize their role as teacher. "Patients need to know what to do on a day-to-day basis, such as what precautions to take depending on their condition," says Carol (Harmon) Mahoney. "We see patients only one or two times a week now. I try to point out things. For the people not cooperating, I would tell them what the choices are and explain that they would need to work on their own. I use a reality-oriented approach. For example, with the head-injured patient, I would use fewer explanations and more encouragement. I would try to be more goal-specific during the session and much more immediate to the patient's needs. I would not do long-term planning. I start out usually asking a lot of questions. I do a thorough evaluation. My approach depends on the patient's age and work and in general who the person is. I adjust the approach by how the person is responding to his or her environment."

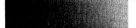

Exploring and Interpreting Motives As Well As Occupation-Based Meanings

In institutional settings, such as a hospital, occupational therapists are challenged to educate themselves about what is meaningful to the patient. The usual symbols of a person's accomplishments, life roles, and community, such as work and leisure interests, spiritual and sexual orientations, are mostly absent. This requires the therapist to take an active role in exploring the connection between how the patient is functioning in the intervention setting with life and relationships outside the medical, service environment.

Providing meaning to what a patient is experiencing is something occupational therapists are always ready to do. "The patient needs to gain the trust that you know what is in the chart, but not by direct means," says Regina Doherty, "such as being able to say to a patient, 'I know what you have just gone through . . . and the reason is that . . .' This is validating, saying why something has happened, when other clinicians do not, and then educating the patient about it. Our role is to connect the medical with the functional."

The content of therapy sessions has a natural progression. "An ideal interaction between me and the patient," says Mike Miller, "would be one in which, in a short period of time, I have gained insight into this person's limitations and, more important, his or her goals and wishes and can place them in the context in which he or she lives. That's in session number 1, or 2, or 3. That's probably reasonable. The next session, creatively, collaboratively, I would use that information to design a treatment program that helps the person regain skills that he or she needs to achieve the goals."

The challenge of interactive therapy, say occupational therapists who were interviewed, is to keep in mind that each person is unique. "It may sound simplistic, but each patient is a real individual, and there is research that must be done about the person," says Jennifer Saylor. "You need to look into the person's roles and psychosocial concerns, to be able to say: 'This is the person.' We look at how the person was functioning before. We need to focus on 'What does the person want to do'? For example, I have had patients who have said, 'I just want to get on and off the toilet.' Then I will explore the emotional aspects of doing this in the hospital. I look at the person's nonverbal communication, the lag time in the conversation. I will then explore the meaning of the problem or disability. Another red flag is when people say, 'I don't like being touched.' Now I am getting more information about the person and what his or her needs are."

Many experienced therapists say that while occupational therapy theory informs their practice, it does so in general, underlying ways rather than in specific how-to ways. Julie Taberman describes her interactive reasoning and maturation as a therapist. "In school, when we learned the frames of reference, I viewed theory as heuristic devices to get us to think about the patient. Now, I get the patients to tell me about their lives. I think about what sorts of things they are missing by being here and about the things that they can do in the hospital with their limitations. For example, things that might get the person to sit up are cooking a meal or playing with the dog. I try to think, 'What will motivate the person?' and 'What will get the person to go home?' We try to do client-centered therapy here, but it is difficult because often the patient says, 'I want to walk,' 'I want to go up the stairs.' It is really difficult to get people to say what they want because they get tired out—they are depressed and institutionalized."

INTERVIEWING EFFECTIVELY

Therapists say the best interactive reasoning involves good interviewing skills. "What I try to find out when we move more toward occupation," says Michael Davison, "is the reason the patient is here. For people who say they don't know, I ask, 'Did you ever know anyone with this problem? If so, how did it affect them?'

My coworker Linda McGettigan came up with this question. I start by investigating patients' knowledge of disease processes, if they are able to articulate them. I ask, 'What is important to you in your daily routine?' Then I ask about the more medical information: if they have any numbness, about things like whether they can manipulate the buttons on their clothes. I usually gather a lot of information in ten minutes, and this of course depends on patients' communication ability. It is very important for them to realize the impact of trauma. If there was aphasia, I would ask a family member. I start with the interview and then use more structure, such as standardized assessments. Usually I use ordinary words like, 'What is important to you?' rather than, 'What do you value?' I do not use abbreviations. I explain the terms. A lot of education goes on."

Educating the client is important because clients need to know the purpose of the activity, or how it is relevant to them, says Janet Kahane. "This way, you give them options and a rationale. I always try to tie in why the activity is useful. If it is in a group setting, I explain the purpose. First, I educate patients about options. I might go over the group schedule and explain how it ties into their needs and what might be most helpful to them. Second, I use techniques of confrontation, reality testing, and validating, such as, 'This is not helpful for you.' Third, I try to use warmth and humor. And fourth, I don't *think* theory, I *embody* theory! It is integrated; it is a part of me. Students do not know how much to push patients. It is important to get a person's history. It helps. I know how much to push someone relative to a diagnosis; I use a different approach, by being either more directive or shorter in directions. Knowing the diagnosis definitely influences how I approach patients. I can adapt to what they can incorporate or process at the time. When I am engaging them, I am analyzing activities to decide what to provide. The other thing is checking with the patient to see if this is okay."

Other therapists agree that it is difficult to put a label on how they practice. "I think if there is any theory or frame of reference I use, it is the model of human occupation, which emphasizes habits and interests," says Liz Freeman. "Using this approach, you ask the question, 'What gets in the way of what you want to do or need to do?'"

GETTING THE WHOLE PICTURE

"A lot of times when I am co-treating, like with the physical therapist, I tend to be blunt and honest," says Dan Kerls. "I sometimes say, 'You are not meeting your goals, you are not safe to go home.' A lot of times I try to sit at eye level and go over the examples I have seen. It is somewhere in between theory and intuition. After a while, it is just in you! I think about the many theories on role and role dysfunction. I see how important their own roles are to the patients and then I empathize with the patients. What is going on is somewhere between reality-testing, expressing empathy, and looking at what roles the patient values.

"I ask the person about his or her past or hobbies to get a better sense of who the person is," continues Kerls. "I am trying to look at the whole picture. I am looking at what the family is doing and whether there is going to be community support for this patient. First, I ask the patient, and then I reality-test with the family, to see if it is accurate. Sometimes, I do that with the family there. Many times, I explain we are going to see how the patient would do something to see how he or she would do it at home. I might introduce a compensatory technique and adaptive equipment while I am doing the other things. With the shorter stay, it hones your ability to prioritize the biggest deficit and what needs to be addressed first. I learned to do this in part by already knowing it, in part from mentors, and in part in my occupational therapy class, by having to identify what was meaningful to me."

Protocols establish the minimum of what is expected from a health care provider. "Therapists have clear expectations of what should be done," says Pat Keck. "These are all part of written competencies for therapists. From the moment they go into the room, they know what they are going to do, such as wash their hands in front of the patient before they shake hands. We have modeled our program after the physician's model, as well as to measure competence. Occupational therapists use clinical reasoning. They go to the chart to find out prior tests and measures and the latest progress notes about what to expect. This is in a ten-minute chart review. This is their clinical reasoning. They should have some strategy when they go into the room and be able to adjust it. For example, if the patient is unable to cooperate, the therapist will make a decision about that based on the chart information. If the patient refuses, the therapist will tell him his rights. It would depend upon the patient's diagnosis. It may be interacting with the family and performing the screen or protocol in a specific way if the patient cannot cooperate. It is the clinical reasoning and the judgement that are variable."

BEING PREPARED

"Therapists need to be able to work with the acute nature of the setting," continues Keck. "The clinical reasoning is very much solid preparation, as is medical knowledge. The occupational therapy knowledge of psychosocial issues is very important because this component of the care might have been overlooked because of the need to stabilize the patient medically. You cannot even move a person's arm without knowing the medical consequences. When interviewing new staff, we always ask therapists about their frames of reference. We are looking for an understanding about occupational performance first. The therapists understand that that is very important here, because that is their role. I think they do use models of occupational performance, such as the neurodevelopmental theory, Rood, or Bobath. Those [models] pale by comparison to the model of human occupation. They use the theory as the basis, the core values behind what they do. The professional part is the deductive reasoning: the review of the record, the patient, knowing the universe of other patients with the diagnosis, consulting with the team or the clinical coordinator, all to guide this reasoning."

The most skillful therapists not only do what they need to medically but also are in touch with the person and his or her life, say therapists. "Even if it is a temporary disease," says Deborah Slater, "they know what the person's life was like before its onset. What is involved is sizing up the situation. You have to think fast and on your feet. It is one thing I do with the staff; I ask them, 'What if they say this, what will you do?' A typical question from a patient is, 'What do I need OT for? All I want to do is walk.' I tell my staff to think about how they would respond. Experienced OTs find strategies that they know are effective. I ask the question, 'What is the most important thing you want to do when you get home?' These are the components that need to be addressed, but in the context of the person. You need to ask only a few questions and not hide behind the evaluation or checklist. It takes maturity, and I am not convinced it can be taught. Either you get it or you don't. For young therapists, it is very difficult. They do not have life experience. Older therapists can more easily tolerate working with patients whose values are different from theirs. Therapists need to have the right questions that can draw people out. That is the main strategy."

LISTENING

Active listening is a skill valued by occupational therapists. Its prominence as a therapeutic tool has been underplayed or even concealed until its recent reemergence under the venue of client-centered therapy. The therapist listens for both what is manifest or being said and what is latent or not being said by the client and family members.

Interactive reasoning is intuitive and requires people skills and knowing how to relate to individuals, therapists emphasize. "It is sort of knowing and being able to deal with the dynamics of people," says Regina Doherty, "being guided by knowing when to do something. For example, if someone was in tears, that would guide my actions. I use my people skills and my intuition to ask myself, 'Am I going to do what I have to do, or am I going to deal with the situation now and come back later for the rest?' To be able to bond with the patient requires experience. You really have to have good observational skills, because that is what guides everything else."

Acting intuitively is not something therapists learn automatically. "I start weighing and sorting through my instincts," says Mike Miller. "One set of my instincts has to do with the physical aspects of the plan. What are the nuts and bolts of the plan? The other is the psychological. What is this person really telling me and how does it affect the relationship so far? I am looking for where are we going. In order for something to have changed, there must be certain factors, and what are those? For example, I feel comfortable reevaluating for discharge placement and discharge date. I use reflection to guide what I say. I use mirroring behaviors and tone of voice. Resistance is a tough one for me. I am starting to learn some principles. What it comes down to is trying to get the patient's perspective and knowing where the person wants to go. You can fall into traps by having your own agenda. I use a client-centered approach. In most cases, I feel that if someone feels you are on their wavelength, then that works. You have to modulate what you do to what is going on with patients by active listening and observing. Your job is to assist them to achieve their goals. Not your goals, *their* goals. There should be a meaningful attachment to the activity."

LOOKING INWARD

Some therapists question whether or how much the current health care environment allows for the use of interactive reasoning. "For me, interactive reasoning is a pushing away of the current health system," says Jennifer Saylor. "It is my value and my wish to help people because they are in a helpless position. My own adversity to the perspective of the current health care system has pushed me to examine why I am in this career. This is more an emotional process than a clinical one. I found that I was becoming mechanical and bored. I believe the questioning has beefed up my clinical skills by knowing more about the patient. The task force OT 2000 [a New England Sinai Hospital and Rehabilitation Center

Occupational Therapy Department committee] has helped me to look at intro-spection. This is in agreement with the philosophy. I spent several years as a COTA at a facility with a lot of severely head-injured patients. It was my per-sonal objective to look at the subtleties of the person. Seeing how bad life situa-tions can be has shown me how things can be mendable. I am a very compassionate person. This is what OT is for me. On the one hand, I abhor com-ponent land; on the other, I respect it."

Objectifying clients according to their diagnosis is the antithesis of good client care, say therapists. "The best interactive reasoning practice I notice for myself and hear from other therapists," says Linda McGettigan, "involves putting my expectations aside. Then I think I am listening to the patient. If I go in and think, 'This patient is a hip and is going to be here two weeks,' then I am not lis-tening to what *she* wants to achieve. It may be that the family is assisting the per-son and that may not be an area I need to address. At that point, after assessing the patient, I usually make a phone call to the family to see if the goals are appro-priate. A lot of times we are not aware that the patient is in a dependent role in the family. Listening is an active process. What I am doing is looking for cues from the patient. If I feel the patient is agreeable to the approach, I am looking for a sign of validation such as enjoyment."

Understanding and Use of Narrative/Symbolic

The occupational therapist who is a skilled practitioner uses ordinary language and stories when talking with clients. By using a familiar reference, the interac-tion has greater impact in establishing the feeling of being understood. When clients feel validated, they are also experiencing a sense of control over their life occupations and interactions.

More advanced practitioners often bring up the use of narrative or the sym-bolic through an interaction or a story. They will state the observations in the context of the client and mirror the clinical observation for the client. "Often, people don't really care, especially with neurological impairment; they have lost so much control, they just don't care," says Regina Doherty. "If you can, you try to give them back a piece of the control and awareness through their own obser-vations. Good therapists can empathize; they can give back control. For example, you can show empathy by saying something like, 'I know you are really frustrated because your arm can't do what you want it to do.' The bonding occurs because the patient thinks, 'She really understands, and she can help me.' People feel ob-ligated to accept what is offered to them—information—but it does not *do* any-thing for them. It really doesn't change the situation. The information is one more thing that they have accepted, but they don't have control of it. They can-not un-herniate a disk. But by giving choices and helping them understand how something will impact their function, you give them back control. It is also very much about timing."

Therapists say it is important to use common sense when they first ap-proach a client. "Some patients want to relate in an intellectual way, and crack-ing jokes may turn off the person," says Deborah Slater. "When you go into a room, you form an image based on a few facts. You may need to do it differently. Some therapists go in like Gangbusters, for example, starting with, 'I am going to tell you. . . .' Depending on the patient, you cannot talk too much, and you cannot roll over them. You have to ask a few well-chosen questions and have a few responses as to how you size up the situation. If the therapist shows incredible compassion, it is a very effective strategy. Use of mental imagery, by asking, 'Tell me about your day, what you do' is also very effective. Then the person knows what occupational therapy is."

BACK TO IDENTITY

The chapter opened with a piece about developmental phases of identity as told by someone who is post-traumatic head injury. To better understand the issues for caregivers and clients, these phases can be conceptualized as pre-injury, hospitalization, and post-injury-healing. The occupational therapist can apply this schema to better understand interactive reasoning along the continuum of care from the hospital to outpatient services and then back to the community.

SUMMARY

The impact of the environment is clearly shown in the hospital and outpatient settings. Occupational therapists employ all of the interactive reasoning strategies described earlier to engage clients in occupational therapy intervention. Without a doubt, these practitioners value a collaborative relationship. They are invested in altering the environment as much as possible to connect with clients in a meaningful way. To this end, they throw away old behaviors and ways of thinking that are nonproductive in practice.

REFLECTIVE QUESTIONS

- What is unique about the institutional setting of a hospital or clinic in terms of service delivery and the client-therapist relationship? Reflect upon your own experience receiving care in a hospital or in assisting someone you cared about in such a situation. Tell the story of your experience.
- Consider your own history as a child, patient, or student when you were in a dependent role. How might your experiences color your relationship with clients and their families in a hospital or clinic environment?
- What type of information do you tend to value, for example, medical versus psychological. How does this influence your hypotheses about client's needs?
- To establish a connection with clients, therapists report using non–therapy-based conversation. What are your areas of interest? Are they broad or narrow? For example, do you know a lot about sports and nothing about world news or the financial world? In what ways can you augment this information through experience or secondary sources?

INFORMATION CHECKPOINTS

4.1. PROCESSES OR STRATEGIES USED BY EXPERIENCED THERAPISTS (ROBERTSON, 1999)

- Pattern matching: A process "where experts access well-organized networks of knowledge in long-term memory. Novices do not have this type of memory to call on so they will use more analytical methods of problem solving which rely on developing a range of possible solutions and hypothesis generation. This is a slower process but is also used by experts in situations that are complex with unique characteristics" (p. 22).
- Clustering: "Clustering related information together is a method used by experts to organize knowledge for easy recall so when they look at an apparently complicated situation they are able to represent it in terms of a small number of patterns or chunks" (p. 24). The therapist gathers information to form a mental image of the situation. "Before meeting the client, the skilled problem solver will have a set of probing questions organised so that the situation can be defined and surrounding issues understood" (p. 25).
- Cues and pattern recognition: Robertson believes that "cues and pattern recognition are significant for effective decision making" (p. 29). She also sees making choices and choosing the hypothesis that best fits as important.

CRITICAL CASE QUESTIONS

4.1.   In her story, Alice says, "I discovered I was in a long process of learning how to take care of myself." Imagine the impact of suddenly being in the hospital and totally dependent on others for your care. How might the hospital context affect someone in Alice's situation?

4.2.   What concerns are raised about identity in Alice's story that may influence her self-image and occupational roles as patient and former patient?

4.3.   What does Alice tell you about the parenting she received as a child, the impact of this history on her self-perceptions before and after the head injury, and the positive gains she had made?

4.4.   What are some clusters or patterns of information in Alice's story related to the impact of her role as patient?

KEY TERMS

BODY LANGUAGE

The nonverbal cues therapists see in how a person physically appears, moves, smells, and sounds.

CLUSTERING OR CHUNKING

The process of putting together small pieces of related information later useful for hypothesis generation.

PROTOCOL

A standardized format often used to gather information or structure interventions.

SCHOOL

5

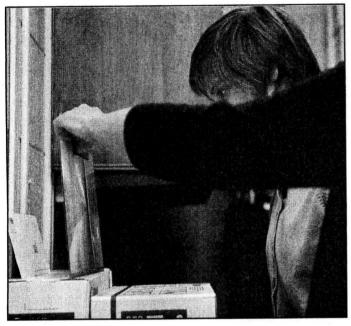

FIGURE 5.1   Validating through Clarifying

VICTOR PLAYS COOL GAMES
By Sharon Ray
March 3, 2000

Victor is seven years old and in the first grade. He was referred to occupational therapy because of clumsiness during fine motor tasks and difficulty with tasks involving the use of scissors or a pencil. He often complained that his hands hurt and seldom completed his written work. Victor's special education team decided that occupational therapy would be appropriate to support his participation in classroom activities. Victor's mother says that Victor did not know why he was being tested but was concerned about being singled out in the class.

When Victor's occupational therapist comes to take him to her room, his best friend Joshua asks where he is going. He says, "I'm going to play some cool games with Sharon. It's fun. Do you want to come?"

OVERVIEW

*T*his chapter includes examples from a variety of school settings and age groups. The therapist is placed in interactive situations in settings that are one-on-one for children with special needs and those situations in which students are seen in integrated classrooms.

It has been recognized that clinical reasoning is important to making decisions on provision of occupational therapy services in the schools (Hall, Robertson, & Turner, 1992). It is assumed that "school-based occupational therapists are concerned with dysfunction and disease only in the context of their effect on the student's capacity to meet educational goals" (p. 929). Nevertheless, as Case-Smith (1997) observes, the literature on the role of promoting psychosocial functioning in school-based practice is "conspicuously absent" (p. 144).

SCHOOL AS CONTEXT

Although it shares similarities with other settings, school-based occupational therapy presents a unique context for interactive reasoning. The school is where the child spends a good part of the day and develops an identity as a student. Endless situations arise where the student builds on this perception of self as a success or a failure. Through school experiences, children learn to incorporate interactions and dealings with others into their world. All of this provides a potentially powerful and influential opportunity for positive interaction with a trained and sensitive person, the occupational therapist. Activity analysis and adaptation are central to thinking about the interactive domain. Developmental theory often underlies the reasoning and techniques selected.

The child's occupational medium is play. In the school setting, the ideal of introducing, using Csikszentmihalyi's (1975) term, the *just right challenge*, or match, is often reported as a goal in play or for being playful. Whereas with other age groups, developmental needs are sometimes overlooked or underestimated, school-based therapists are giving these issues their rightful emphasis. For example, the therapists are tacitly drawing upon Mosey's (1970) developmental group model in adapting a classroom group activity by bringing other children into an activity with the child with special needs, and vice versa. Inclusion theory, friendship theory, and other points of view are also implied in the manner to which they structure interactions and activities. The developmental theories from psychology and occupational therapy, reviewed in chapter 1, appear to strongly influence therapists' reasoning in the schools.

In the chapter opening case study, the student appears uncomfortable with his need for help. The child's mother reports that Victor was concerned about being singled out in class. Victor's natural instinct is to want to play and be involved with others as usual. The school-based therapists describe strategies that address the child's self-esteem needs and developmentally appropriate occupational interests, such as play. (See Critical Case Questions 5.1 and 5.2.) The interventions require a high degree of involvement and multiple strategies. The therapists working in schools who were interviewed describe a practice with

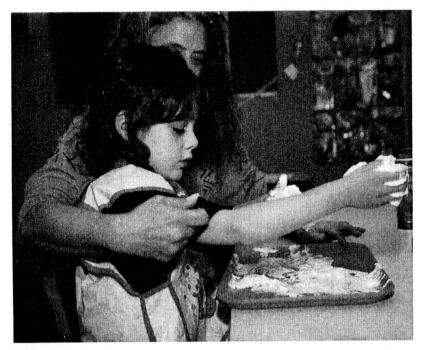

FIGURE 5.2 Active Collaboration through the Just Right, Occupation-Based Challenge

complex issues and multiple use of interactive reasoning concepts and techniques. Some of the approaches they discussed include providing choices, being client centered, focusing on the child, focusing on fun, building trust, and respecting style differences.

ACTIVE PARTICIPATION AND COLLABORATION

Without the child's active involvement in occupational therapy, the intervention process is doomed. As in the case of Victor in the opening scenario, the school-based therapist typically looks for points of choice in the very ordinary activities of the child. The therapist must make judgements, act spontaneously, and accept what at times seems like very modest gains. The following examples illustrate the therapist's role in establishing a collaborative relationship with not only the student but also the student's extended family and friendship system, as well as other teachers or resources within the school.

PROVIDING CHOICES

One of the hallmarks of an experienced occupational therapist is that the practitioner provides the client an opportunity to make choices around treatment. This is a goal even if the client has limitations, says Molly Campbell, OTR/L, of the Brookline Public Schools and the Perkins School for the Blind. On the other hand, the provision of choices lets therapists learn about their clients and their goals by observing their decision-making process. "If I am having a hard time naturally relating to the person, I would collaborate with others to see if [the problem] is in my technique, fearing that it is my personality. This is less mature than asking whether I am using the right approach. It might be a pattern with the student; for example, does the student need a break rather than just to focus on the task?"

Being attuned to the specific needs of the client is a requirement despite the child's diagnosis or age. Therefore, occupational therapists must be adept at changing approaches or goals as a case calls for it, often without warning. "Our emphasis is in wheeled mobility and adaptive seating and positioning," says Gary Rabideau, OTR/L, of the Massachusetts Hospital School. "That is our niche, or expertise. Often the project or referral is around functional mobility. It may be a family or therapist who refers for modification or a solution regarding equipment for mobility. There is the mechanical piece, but it all begins with assessing the person." While the most relevant input on what a student needs most comes from discerning cues directly from the child, important information comes from the child's teacher or principal, others in the school, and the child's parents or caregivers. The source of information might be the family member, primary therapist, or a larger group of people.

BEING CLIENT CENTERED

Rabideau usually co-leads the interview process with a partner who is a physical therapist. "A lot of the process is the dynamic between me, the therapist, and the individual. If we are talking about existing or new-wheeled mobility, we are trying to assess the client's functional goals. The person's goals, needs, and interests are important from the beginning. If the motivation or incentive is not with the client, the equipment goes unused. The exchange is very client centered when things are going well."

Rabideau identified three areas of information that guide the process of determining appropriate equipment as well as the person's goals and interests:

1. *Medical-physical status* involves linking physical abilities and cognitive-perceptual status to the ability to use equipment. The input of others is sought here.
2. *Functional status* involves everything from the ADL [activities of daily living], to vocation, avocation, ability to transfer, and mobility status.
3. *Environmental factors* include types of environments, settings, transportation needs, the work site, and recreational environment.

PROBLEM SOLVING

Even in optimal circumstances, occupational therapists have to use all their skills as clinicians to adapt to the circumstances in which they find themselves. In a school setting, says Debra Plugis, OTR/L, of the Framingham Public Schools, many children have multiple needs. "Many of the students have behavioral problems. My work involves observing, using theory, and acting. For example, one child really bossed me around. I had to accommodate and stretch the extra mile so she would learn to trust me. My job is to do what I can do to help the child reach her therapeutic goals. It might not be a big stupendous thing. It could be simply gaining mutual cooperation."

"In my pediatrics practice, I see many kids with sensory integration problems," says Laura (Guertin) Impemba, OTR/L, of Healthsouth Braintree Pediatric Rehabilitation in Melrose. "It is very important to get the cues with this population. It may be disastrous to be overly bubbly with children with sensory integration problems. It is essential to establish the mood. The sensory issues are essential to any work with these kids, whether it be muscle tone or some other concern. It involves sensing whether they need sensory stimulation or calming so they can maintain focus. Some kids come in literally bouncing, and if I am too energetic, it would feed into their hyperarousal. I try to decrease the amount of stimulation they have to deal with, and this helps to calm them, for example, by talking softly, lowering the lights, and putting the child in a swing. Your first step is judging where this child is today, because it can change from day to day. Then, you have to figure out how to bring the child to an adequate level of arousal through observation, modifying my type of interaction, for example, voice modulation, and adapting the environment and the activity. This is all based on sensory integrative theory, but now I know the effects without thinking about it."

Similarly, Merrill Forman, OTR/L, of the Brookline Public Schools, uses theory to guide and inform her therapy. She describes her job in terms of finding the just right challenge. "I think in terms of the activity and the relationship between the child, the activity, and me. I usually base what I do on the goals for the child and developmentally where the child is. I also judge whether the activity is the just right challenge. Is it pushing the child a bit where he or she can grow? I see how the child is that day and make a decision. I consider whether the child was sick the day before or not or had slept well. I read the situation at the moment and make a decision as to what would work best at the time."

ENGAGING/CONNECTING AND CREATING A HOLDING ENVIRONMENT

Engaging and connecting with a child requires therapists to put aside their own needs and genuinely accept the student's individuality. To create a holding environment, the therapist must be fully present at the child's level of need. Only then can the therapeutic process take place. If the student is thirsty, for example, the therapist provides or helps the child quench that thirst. If the student needs the therapist to be like a teacher, the therapist acts within the child's stereotype and may become didactic and an authority figure. Similarly, if the child needs a therapist as playmate, the practitioner interacts playfully.

In the school setting, children with disabilities can find themselves in situations where they both experience hurtful behavior and are overly protected by teachers or peers. It is critical that the student perceive tender acceptance from the therapist to avoid the possibility of further humiliation and damage to a weakened self-image. The negative attitude of others easily attaches itself to the parts of an already fragile ego. The therapist must stand for a consistent figure of acceptance—for the student is more than likely feeling damaged.

PROVIDING A SAFE ENVIRONMENT

In schools where achievement is the valued commodity, the student requires an occupational therapy environment where corrective, positive experiences are abundant to protect the child against further unsatisfying interpersonal, social, and academic experiences. The therapists in the following examples candidly describe the challenges of connecting with children and creating a holding environment in the school setting.

Molly Campbell finds that the key to effective therapy is to relate to the client on a human, and humane, level. "Get into the person. Adapt the activity, interaction, and equipment to match the person. Tell yourself the puzzle is not solved yet—don't get discouraged when you are trying, but rather, realize that you have a huge puzzle."

Timing and freshness are critical components to success, contends Campbell. "There is the reinforcement of more kindness and enthusiasm. There is genuinely appreciating the person, accepting the person, and just being there and celebrating the success. Some people forget that [therapy] is about the person with the disability and it is *not* about themselves. It is absolutely about the person with the disability."

FOCUSING ON THE CHILD

Debbie Caruso agrees. "I love my job and I love my kids. The flip side is when I cannot connect with a child or a family. It is very hard for me. When I cannot connect with a child, I *do* take it personally. But with time I have learned it is not about me."

If the focus is on the person with the disability, then treatment will be possible when the client values the activity being done. "I think something that helps the process is to look at control," says Gary Rabideau. "One thing we find here is that if our students—the clients—have a connection to their piece of equipment, then it goes well. Finding a motivator with the person and the piece of equipment is essential. We work that angle hard if the person is having trouble. We connect the value of the equipment to the person in doing a valued activity. The client is controlling the process. Whereas the physical therapist leads more of the motor elements, I conduct the cognitive process, the connection between the person and the means for the person to do something that is important to him or her. For example, you might want to start by asking what color toy the child wants so the child will get some ownership. We try to put the attention on the equipment and the value to the child. One of the concerns I have about young therapists is that they can be too controlling. Sometimes, they try to dictate to the client and are not client-centered. It is almost too easy to be parental and overdriving, and it is really important that the therapy process be client driven."

FOCUSING ON FUN

Occupational therapists who work with children underscore that therapy must also be about having fun. "Therapy can be scary for children," says Laura Snell, OTR/L, of the Bay Cove Early Intervention Center in Dorchester. "With the child, there are certain moments in the therapy session when you are trying to make things fun. You are doing things to meet goals, yet it is spontaneous fun, noncontrived. It never, ever works if you say it is going to be this or that. It is looking at what the child is doing and determining how best to incorporate this."

Debra Plugis agrees. "Best practice occurs when there is a natural and smooth flow of things happening, where I can sense that I can push the children a little more or expect more. I can have them try new things. A lot of the children are resistant to the therapy aspect of it, especially the older ones. I have to make it fun." However, that is not always appropriate. "Sometimes it is pointless to make it fun. I point out that this is like medicine you have to take. For example, I work with some children with low tone who find it very hard to write. I may have to charm them, but they still have to do the work. Other children with sensory integration problems might only want to jump. You try to make treatment fun and interesting.

"Each child is an individual," continues Debra Plugis. "I work with what the personality means to me and shape the relationship and activity so there is a high level of interest and it is not boring, and the child wants to work. I feel that I can be a playful partner, yet also serious, and some of the playful part is really good for them. A laid-back, easy personality works for one child and not for another. It is not that I go around changing my personality, but limit setting can be effective with one child and not the next. You just have to switch speed and gears. You have to develop the relationship."

WHEN IT DOESN'T WORK

Part of being a professional is recognizing when treatment is not being effective because of a clash of personalities. "Certain aspects of my personality change to accommodate to the child, yet my basic personality doesn't change," says Debra Plugis. "That is why I like to work with other therapists. For example, one child was out of control, and I asked another therapist to take over the case. To be blunt about it, the child and I just rubbed each other the wrong way. He worked great with someone else. They had a better personality fit."

BUILDING TRUST

In addition to having a playful spirit, a therapist must be able to build trust with a young client. "I think it takes a lot of skill to work with the preschool age group," says Merrill Forman. "You need to be really upbeat and flexible. I use a lot of drama and emotion in my work, especially with children diagnosed with a pervasive developmental disability [PDD], such as autism, to get them motivated and to connect with them. You need to get them to relate to you physically. For example, I sit on the floor and make eye contact at their level. I bring in materials to help connect with them. I use materials in a way to really spark their interest and connection, for example, a crayon in a sparkly box. That is not an ordinary crayon, and it may motivate the child to take an interest in using it. It is about taking time to build up trust and a connection. I also use the typically developing children in the classroom. I work with them and I do an activity for the whole class. Then the child I plan to work with may want to join the pack."

Couching all activities in play is essential to reaching children at their level, says Sharon Ray, OTR/L, of the Boston School of Occupational Therapy at Tufts University. "Whether or not a child knows he or she has a problem, it is critical to preserve the child's self-esteem. In the developmental process where the child is, therapeutic play is the medium of play. Therapists should give children ways of marking their progress and ownership in a way that they understand."

Ray also advises therapists to think about what children value and what they consider important as their occupation. "The key is reading the child, the child's interpretation, going where the child is and making the child aware of what he or she can accomplish, and adding to it," says Ray. "It is always important that children feel good about what they can do. Your role as a therapist is to find what they can do. Sometimes it is trial and error; that is, the interaction is based upon the reasoning until they have ownership. It is a way of looking at the child and finding out what the next step is."

Therapists know that their treatment is working when a client takes the initiative in therapy. "The way I feel and know a good interaction is when children open up," says Debbie Caruso. "They start to share information about things that happen at home or things that happen at school; they want me to be part of their life. They show they have established trust. That is also true with siblings and with teachers who want to share their classroom with me. On the flip side, if a teacher does not want to know something, it is an equally powerful signal that something is not right, and I need to find out what is going on. There are different levels of interaction. Some are very pleasant, and some are more difficult."

EXPLORING AND INTERPRETING MOTIVES AS WELL AS OCCUPATION-BASED MEANINGS

Case-Smith (1997) studied therapists' stories that describe successful school-based practice. She found that "strategies that emphasized personal interaction and meaningful activities were used to help students achieve success." (See Critical Case Question 5.3.) "In conditional reasoning, the occupational therapist attempts to understand the problem or disability from the student's perspective. Important to this process is establishing a relationship with the student (i.e., interactional reasoning) and then individualizing therapy to the student's own interests or goals" (p. 145). (See Information Checkpoint 5.1.) The following is a sample of what therapists said about motivation through occupation-based meaning.

"I try to find out the child's and the family's interests in order to make the activity meaningful," says Debbie Caruso. "For example, I have a child who wants to always make everything into a train activity. If I use a train, he will get involved in the activity."

"I think in the end I always go back to theory," says Debra Plugis. "Are they acting this way because they have a sensory integration problem, or a behavior problem, or something else? You have to have the big picture. Not that they *are* a disability but that they have a personality. This approach also applies to working with parents."

THE LARGER PICTURE

"I work a lot with teachers to see what they are working on in order to relate what I am doing to what the class is doing," says Merrill Forman. "I may also give the teacher a project to work on that would meet my child's needs. I observe what the child is doing when I come into the classroom. In addition, I can modify my intent to do something one-on-one by working with two children who might be playing. That way, I could use the materials the children are using and modify them to meet the therapeutic goal. This requires being spontaneous and modifying circumstances to see where the child is. It is easy to flow into what is happening in preschool and later years when you are more in a supporting role. The children are really playing, and you concentrate on the therapy."

Therapists need to reach out to teachers in a way that is respectful of their role in the school setting yet acknowledges how they can work with the other team members to help the child. "You also want to empower teachers," says Sharon Ray, OTR/L, Boston School of Occupational Therapy at Tufts University in Medford. "First, listen to where they are. Understanding is then empowering them by allowing them to do what they want. Empowering a child is very different. It depends upon age of child and should be kept within the context of play. The therapist must try to follow the child's cues and attempt to be where the child is—tying it in with what is familiar and usual for the child—because otherwise the child thinks he or she is bad. Go to where the child is; go to the child's level, for example, at eye level and on the floor. Empower children, and involve them so they know how to do for themselves." (See Information Checkpoint 5.2.)

LISTENING

Therapist listening involves observation of verbal and nonverbal cues. Eye contact is often mentioned as important to listening. However, the resultant intensity of the gaze—the amount and type of attention, whether it is verbal or visual—versus tactile input, for example, is modified according to the individual child's needs and tolerance. In the following, two therapists capture what others also said about the value of listening and making eye contact.

"With children it is good to just be an observer and see what they are about rather than see later and be surprised," says Debra Plugis. "I like to see what kind of personality they have. Do they need a lot of attention? Are they rigid and bossy? Finding those things up front really helps."

"The main thing I try to establish is eye contact," says Debbie Caruso. "In addition, I try as often as I can to contact the teacher if I am having a difficult time. I try to find ways to have the child open up."

UNDERSTANDING AND USE OF NARRATIVE/SYMBOLIC

It is especially difficult for students with special needs to negotiate the different cultural worlds of their community, family, classroom, and therapy (Mattingly & Beer, 1995). Understanding the symbolic elements communicated by students of a variety of cultural backgrounds is necessary to successful interventions. Such understanding requires occupational therapists to learn about diverse and multiple cultures that include not only race and ethnicity but also families, workplaces, institutions, classes and neighborhoods, and professions (Mattingly & Beer, 1995).

Metaphors and metaphorical techniques are suggested as a means to provide options that the child might not be aware of (Fazio, 1992). According to Fazio, "For some children, it is necessary to provide a metaphor to define the problem in a personal way" (p. 114). She suggests storytelling, along with guided affective imagery, as a treatment approach to help the child or adolescent see things differently.

The following are some examples of how therapists employ narrative and the symbolic in their interactive reasoning and actions. They consider the world of the child from the multiple, sometimes conflicting, layers of culture.

"I try to find out things out about the children and about the parents," says Debra Plugis. "Some of the parents are really difficult, and they expect a lot. I try to find out what kind of environment they come from."

"I try to find out what the child is interested in and what the family values are," says Debbie Caruso. "For example, I see one child on Friday afternoons. For that family, the goal is to have their daughter sit through Friday night dinner. I try to find out what interests and motivates the child, the family, and the teacher. I try to find out what the main goal is and try to build that into our interactions."

RESPECTING STYLE DIFFERENCES

"One of the main things," adds Merrill Forman, "is to remember that it is the teacher's classroom and you are really a visitor. It is important to follow the teacher's rules. However, you can apply what you learn from one teacher to another classroom. Figuring out how to work with different styles of teachers can be a challenge. You need to be able to prioritize for each student and teacher which modifications you can realistically implement. I am really working with others to help them be able to water the seed, so to speak. Therefore, working with the various styles is key."

"We elicit images, for example, 'picture yourself at school,' 'picture yourself at work,'" says Gary Rabideau. "We try to be concrete and show them equipment, and when they are very active and are able to put themselves in that piece of equipment, then we are doing a better job."

"SOCIAL STORIES"

"We use social stories with children who have difficulty understanding a social situation," says Debbie Caruso. "A social story is very brief. You write a story about what Johnny would do in a particular situation. You may draw illustrations or take a photograph. For concrete thinkers, we may have to use a social story to have them preview and practice a social situation. You have them work through things and practice in advance. You may elaborate on the story. It looks easy, but it is very complex. The problem-solving aspect is important. I have yet to have an occupational therapy student who could not grasp this concept after a couple of months. Students first concentrate on the physical aspect and then incorporate the emotional."

BACK TO VICTOR

Victor improved in occupational therapy. Through use of problem solving, finding the just-right challenge, and working with his mother, the therapist and child became partners. With the perception of therapy as fun, Victor was able to incorporate the intervention as a positive experience in his developing identity as a student.

SUMMARY

The issues related to interactive reasoning in school-based practice were presented in chapter 5. Strategies supported include involving the student, teacher, and family in the intervention process. The value of using the child's natural play or educational environment as well as understanding the school's and the child's cultures is illustrated. The need to pay special attention to the psychological and emotional aspects of the child is emphasized in the reasoning about interactions and in the process of therapeutic use of self as well as activities in an educational environment.

REFLECTIVE QUESTIONS

- Cultural orientation is an important area of consideration in school-based practice. In one example, a therapist reported that for one family it was important for the child to sit through Friday night dinner. For an orthodox Jewish family, the Friday night Sabbath meal holds important traditions. While it is important to this family, other families may hold other cultural traditions. In this and other situations, how might the cultural orientation of the child, teacher, and school influence interactive reasoning for the occupational therapist?
- What is your own cultural orientation, and how might it influence your interactive reasoning?
- How would you characterize the difference in interactive style between the occupational therapist working in the integrated classroom in an educational setting and one working in a specialized service delivery program such as a clinic or home program? In thinking about your own interactive style, what differences do you perceive in your interactions with a student and family in a school or clinic versus a home environment? Do you or would you like to modify your approach, and why?
- How would you incorporate therapeutic play in your interactive reasoning? If you don't consider yourself playful, what processes can you introduce into your work to enhance this aspect of the therapeutic relationship?
- Imagine the stories of children, parents, and teachers about situations in which they perceived themselves as different. How might these perceptions inform your work as an occupational therapist?

INFORMATION CHECKPOINTS

5.1 VARIABLES RELATED TO SUCCESSFUL SCHOOL-BASED PRACTICE (CASE-SMITH, 1997)

- Reframing the child's problems or behaviors in terms of the key or underlying basis.
- Supporting the child's psychosocial core and self-image.
- Collaboration with team members on important life goals and family support.

5.2 Empowerment

Empowering the child and family builds trust (Sharon Ray).

Critical Case Questions

5.1. Victor invites his friend to join his visit to the occupational therapist. What issues are of concern to Victor, his mother, the special education team, and the occupational therapist?

5.2. As an occupational therapist, what would you do when Victor brings his friend Joshua to your room?

5.3. Knowing the child's feelings about being singled out, how in your interactions and selection of activities can you build upon Victor's presenting a visit to Sharon as fun?

Key Terms

Cultural Orientation

A person's racial orientation, ethnicity, religious orientation, sexual orientation, social-educational class orientation, and orientation to family, workplace, institutions, and neighborhood.

Just Right Challenge

In an activity, the just right, or optimal, challenge leads to satisfaction (Csikszentmihalyi, 1975).

Psychosocial Functioning

A performance component area involving psychological concerns such as self-identity, interests, values, social skills, and such self-management skills as time management and accepting limits.

Sensory Integration

A performance component area involving sensory motor systems that influences the child's ability to carry out school and play activities, for example.

Social Story

A series of activities built around a short story. For example, the activities can include viewing and talking about a photograph or a drawing. The brief story is used to help a child envision a situation more concretely and to preview and practice a social situation (Debbie Caruso).

COMMUNITY

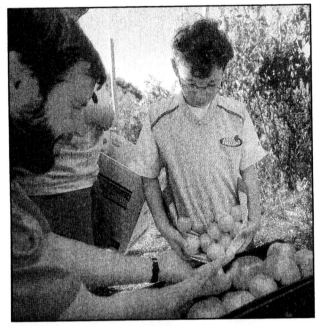

FIGURE 6.1   Stories in the Culture of Community

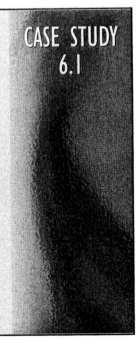

BETTER THAN SEX
By Mike Miller
(February 6, 2000)*

CASE STUDY
6.1

"*I*t's such a rush, man, it's like, better than sex!"

It took me long enough to figure out the system to page my friend in the huge apartment complex. I knew his room number, thanks to my cognitive prosthesis—a little digital voice recorder I confiscated from my technologically unworthy better half. However, dialing the room number got me nowhere. I'll be here forever! Finally, I look on the board next to the phone—the codes are listed (50 of them) by last name, first initial. Great! I call him up and within seconds I'm upstairs knocking on the door. I wonder what it must be like for my buddy, wondering where I was. An explosive greeting

*Originally written in class assignment for Dr. Maureen Fleming, Tufts University, Boston School of Occupational Therapy

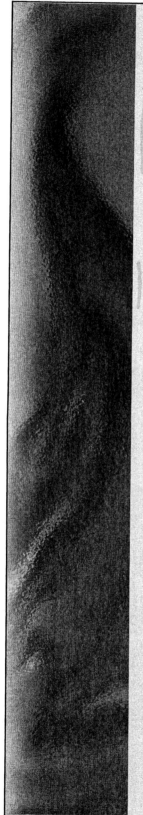

followed in slow motion, I, consciously trying to act cool, he, visibly elated. I silently admonish myself for my ongoing reluctance. It was Friday night, but we had planned this long ago, and I had already canceled once. I tried to relax and remember why I was there: to have a fun time with a valued friend.

Potential crisis number one: what movie theater? It was raining and snowing something fierce and the traffic was piled up everywhere. I am not familiar with this side of town; can I rely on my friend's recall? Where's the closest theater? We decide to risk spontaneity and head for the door, but not before checking out the new exercise treadmill in the main room. This gives me a chance to ask how it is going. "Does that help with the contractures?" I wonder what it must be like for my friend, walking over a curb. I hold his cane while Carlos puts on his jacket, and when we get outside, he asks me to hold on to him because the sidewalk is slippery. "I hope you don't mind if I ask you some questions tonight." Carlos is open and tells me he likes it when people ask questions. I wonder why I thought it would be different for a person with an impairment; everybody likes to talk about himself or herself. Still, I rationalize this by reminding him that what I learn from him can help me with clients I might see with similar symptoms. What I did not know was the depth of the wisdom I would experience that night.

"Drive slow, man. I always take the middle lane; I like the middle lane cause its not too fast and people aren't trying to cut in front of you from the ramps," says Carlos in a pleading tone. I slow from 45 to 40. It is slippery, but I consider myself a cautious driver anyway. I wonder what it must be like for my passenger, being out of control. Everything is a decision. I drop Carlos off at the front, trying to justify treating him differently and trying to remember he is the stronger man. The new Bruce Willis movie is starting shortly, and Carlos pays for the tickets. "You can get the popcorn," he says. We walk through the lobby. I wonder if people notice anything different. I stay focused and navigate through the crowd. "Isn't it that way?" I ask. I'm thinking we're going to have to traipse back and forth down the hall a couple of times, but my friend impresses me again; he knows where we're going. Next decision: where to sit. The theater is crowded enough, and we have to get by people; Carlos likes to sit in the middle. We do our best and find a seat towards the front, necessitating a move by three young women.

It is late when the show gets out, and I learn that Carlos has not eaten. We decide to look for Chinese food, and I decide to probe. "Have you been using your electronic organizer?" Carlos tells me all about the memory aids and the doctors administering more cognitive tests, and nobody believing him when he says he loses his orientation. "I'll be somewhere and just totally forget where I am and what I'm doing. It's scary. The doctors tell me I'm fine, and point to some test scores." He pleads with them to no avail. I remind him as only an OT can that he (Carlos) is the only person who knows about Carlos, and he's his own best doctor sometimes. He goes on to talk about what a liberating experience it was to have half his brains wiped out in an instant. "God had a reason for all this, Mike. I was so unhappy before. I had money, I had women, people always wanted to party with me."

"I'm so happy now," he said, and I wonder what it must be like for my teacher, with his whole life ahead of him. I asked how long he was in a coma, knowing the functional impact length of time has on prognosis. "Seven weeks," he said. "My family was going to take me off life support soon if I didn't come out of it. The doctors wrote me off."

"Look at you now!" was the only response I could muster. I remembered back four years. I was working in a rehab hospital as a therapeutic recreation aide. Carlos was making strides, I had heard, but I did not have much contact with him, except to visit and offer whatever encouragement I could. He had invited my wife and me to his mother's for an authentic Spanish dinner. My policy was not to befriend clients, but he did live just up the street, and it would be a chance to experience a completely new culture . . . "How did Carlos get injured?" I had asked his therapist. "Motorcycle accident." And I wondered what it must be like for our client, with his whole life ahead of him. "Do you think they should be illegal?" I asked. "Yes, a motorcycle wants you to get on it, man. It says—go faster, go faster. And each time you twist the throttle it's another rush. It's such a rush, man, it's like, better than sex!"

OVERVIEW

$\mathcal{F}$ollowing the discussion of school-based practice, this chapter takes us to other community settings where occupational therapists work. It is befitting to conclude this section of the book with an eye to the future. As with hospital and clinic-based practice, as well as the schools, the dynamics of community settings have an impact on interactive reasoning. Attention needs to be paid to multiple narratives or stories: the therapist, the client or the student, the program, the employer or company, and the larger community. (See Critical Case Question 6.1.) (See Information Checkpoint 6.1.)

Community-based practice is considered the future of occupational therapy practice in the United States. Yet the literature on clinical reasoning with a community focus, interactive reasoning in particular, is almost nonexistent. Munroe (1996), who undertook a qualitative study of therapists delivering home care services in Scotland, sought to find out about clinical reasoning in community occupational therapy. She found that decision making was more concerned with interactive reasoning than any other pattern of reasoning. The reasoning was contextual or pragmatic in response to contextual influences of the client and caregiver in the home setting. Respondents in her study used patterns of reasoning, such as reflection in action during home visits, decision making about interactive issues, and reasoning. (See Critical Case Question 6.2.)

One other report of clinical reasoning in community-based practice was reported in the *British Journal of Occupational Therapy*. Fortune and Ryan (1996) discovered a system of caseload management based upon perceived complexity, using Mattingly and Fleming's clinical reasoning framework. They propose that therapists' caseloads can be managed to consist of complex and simple work through an analysis of type and amount of clinical reasoning required.

ACTIVE PARTICIPATION AND COLLABORATION

In the following examples, the procedural aspects of practice directly influence the professional's interactive reasoning. As reflected in the literature, therapists are making decisions about goals and the nature of collaboration with pragmatic concerns in mind. Practicalities may include such things as number of treatment sessions allocated and company expectations. The themes that appear in the conversations with community occupational therapists have to do with such issues as a client-centered approach, building a relationship, sharing goals, providing hope, seeing the big picture, establishing credibility, and "felt sense."

In today's health care environment, therapists are required to know from the start of treatment what the scope will be of their involvement with the client. They must be able to justify to themselves and the client, as well as to the referral source and to third-party payers, what their plan of action will involve and over how long a period.

"I think part of the interaction in acute care is that you have to conceive of one session as *the* session," says Kathy Hanlon, OTR/L, of the Newton Wellesley Hospital. "You need to decide what piece of work out of the whole picture needs to be done. You may have only one or two sessions. You have to be realistic in what you can expect to accomplish. You need to work with the client to decide on goals."

Some therapists see their initial task with the client as identifying goals. "At the beginning, even before I start working with a client, we set an agenda for therapy," says Tom Mercier, OTR/L, of Invacare Corporation New England Region. "If clients cannot participate in this process, I will identify what they need."

Mercier borrows this approach to conceptualizing an interaction from the business world. "I use personal selling skills (PSS), which is an IBM methodology." He identifies several steps to the process:

- set an agenda,
- ask probing questions,
- address objections,
- summarize what is spoken about, and
- come to a decision on how the meeting went.

"This is a goal-based process," says Mercier. "Not, 'this is just what you have to do,' but 'what would you like to accomplish?'"

THE ART OF RELATIONSHIP

A special dynamic takes place when the occupational therapist and the client are in sync, that occurs because the process is well thought out, and doesn't occur simply by chance. "A huge part of what makes me feel that things are going well is that the relationship is a two-way street," says Thayer McCain, OTR/L, of Medford private practice Thriving at Home. "It is important to know that the client is sharing the same goals. For me the flow happens when I can feel the person with me, that he or she is making decisions with me and can challenge me. This happens when the client has heard what I said and comes back with an alternative as to what would work or by dissecting what would or would not work—not just an off-the-cuff statement that this or that would not work. For instance, one man I was working with, who had a spinal cord injury, came up with ideas of his own, and it felt really right. It is a collaborative process where the person is really engaged, as compared to a medical model where the process is more passive."

ENGAGING/CONNECTING AND CREATING A HOLDING ENVIRONMENT

As in the chapter opening case study, therapists talk about what is going on in their heads as they make decisions about what to say and how to direct a conversation. In connection and holding, therapists are matching the interaction with their sense of what the person needs. (See Critical Case Question 6.3.) (See Information Checkpoint 6.2.)

Therapists describe connecting with a client as an active process that is well thought out and therapeutic but at the same time respectful of the client's humanity. "I think there is a real connection in the best interactive practice," says Ellen Cohen Kaplan, OTR/L, who is in private practice and works for Harvard Community Health Plan. "What I am saying resonates with clients. The things I say make sense to them, and I can immediately understand their perspectives from my relationship with them."

While a therapist's behavior is grounded on the theory behind therapeutic practice, the relationship itself may be founded at first on a more intuitive person-to-person level. "I think empathy precedes any type of theory," says Cohen Kaplan. "The first thing I think is, 'How would I want to make the client comfortable?' That is, to validate, to echo back, to paraphrase. For me, empathy is the first rule of thumb. The second is a real comfort level with the material; it can let

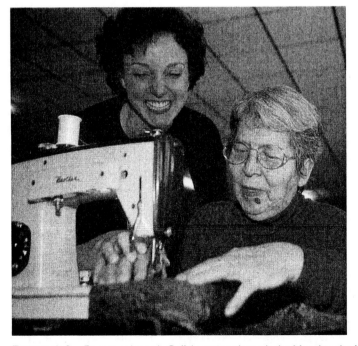

FIGURE 6.2   Engaging through Collaboration through the Mood in the Moment to Moment

me delve further. Being female, I relate much more to what the females say. I keep it very conscious so as not to lose what the men are saying. If I feel I am likely to lose what a client is saying, I try to step out of the situation. I redirect the client. I am analyzing, using metacognitive processes and analysis of counter-transference. For example, as a therapist, you frame it and stay in the moment. I remember that this is not my family member. It is intentional what I say, but not necessarily what I am thinking. If clients can understand what countertransference is and experience it, it can be used, but it depends on how evolved they are."

THERAPEUTIC APPROACH

Cohen Kaplan's therapeutic behavior is driven by the frame of reference. "I use a cognitive behavioral approach. I give homework. You can change how you react by changing how you act. I use psychodynamic object relations theory. I take it slow with someone who is resistant. I make it a point to connect with people. I talk to them about things that have nothing to do with the group. The one-to-one connection makes them feel an unconditional acceptance. It can be around anything. The better your fund of knowledge, the more points to connect, such as about sports or contracting." (See Information Checkpoint 6.3.)

Finding common interests is a step in the process of effective interaction, but to begin the therapeutic relationship, a therapist must be able to empathize with the client. "I think as an occupational therapist, but I am working with the well population," says Kathy Hanlon, OTR/L, of the Newton Wellesley Hospital. "It is important to have a good empathic connection with the client and a real sense of what the person is going through. The therapist sees the person as a real person and not a category. The therapist is asking open-ended questions and making statements like, 'I think this may be a place where you are stuck' and not 'this is your problem.' Always feed the information back to the patient." (See Information Checkpoint 6.4.)

GIFT OF HOPE

In her occupational therapy practice, Cohen Kaplan follows a principle in acute care advanced by Irvin D. Yalom. It is an approach that gives hope to the client. "The relationship is a piece of the whole long-term picture," says Cohen Kaplan. "In acute care, you may not see the person over time, but you are a part of the continuum of care. If you give a person a good enough interaction, he or she may feel well enough to go on. This is not easy to do. If a person is anxious, I might do something with him or her to calm the person down, for example, deep breathing. I would certainly name what the person is going through. I will give hope that the person will not always be where he or she is now."

While connecting with another individual, especially professionally, is not always simple, it can ease the process for therapists to act themselves. Hanlon says, "I might use humor, a little bit of gentle humor, to get the person to smile. Sometimes I use my own feelings. I try to read the person to see if this [anxiety] is coming from him or her. Or is it a negative reaction on my part, as in, is the person hitting my buttons? You need to handle the personal reaction and put this aside if it is coming from you. It needs to be out of the interaction. This quick mental checklist happens in a split second. Do I understand this person's state of mind, knowing that my state of mind might not be the same? I might understand the feeling state, although I am not feeling it at the time. How can we use this approach to help the person? I might teach anxiety management techniques or other skills to help the client deal with what he or she is experiencing."

ESTABLISHING CREDIBILITY

Connecting with a client can start with establishing rapport. "An important element of interactive practice is that I engage the client initially," says Mercier. "For example, when I worked with sales reps, I would tell them their job is the hardest in the company. Then I would say my job is to help them and to make their job easier. I was trying to establish credibility. The other trainers were sales reps, and I wasn't, and I had to establish credibility."

Most therapists say they can tell immediately when they are successful at building a relationship. "The best interactive practice is when I can tell that people are listening to me, that they understand what I am saying," says Tom Mercier. "Sales reps tend to be Type A and aggressive personalities. They often have trouble listening. A good sales rep comes in with a strong agenda, which is to sell. When something is going well, the sales reps are giving me feedback that they see my point. If they are trying to justify themselves, they are not listening."

Good therapists use all of their professional and life experiences in reaching out to clients. "I think that my psych skills are integrated—the personal cues, the therapeutic relationship, and just sensing things to see if I can joke and keep things light. It involves taking one step back," says Thayer McCain. "One of the initial goals is letting patients see that I know their world is different from mine. I try to validate what they are going through from their perspective. I want to let them know that I realize that things are more complex than they seem. An example of that is just validating how disorienting and disruptive it is to be in the hospital for one week. I think therapists ignore that aspect of trying to normalize the situation by not letting the patient know that disorientation is to be expected. I also stress that it is important to let caretakers know that they need to look at their own needs as much as their partner's needs . . . to encourage them to get some respite. It is a holistic approach. That is why I love home care. That is why occupational therapy is suited for home care. There is an organic process in home care. Certainly part of it is a felt sense."

EXPLORING AND INTERPRETING MOTIVES AS WELL AS OCCUPATION-BASED MEANINGS

The community context is by definition occupation-based. Therapists explore the meaning of occupations and try to understand motivation from this perspective. In doing so, the therapist bridges the person's inner world, with the occupation-based problem and intervention, and the larger system such as school, family, and community. This requires maintaining a neutral posture about the perceived value of occupations, as the choices are client centered.

Therapists working in the community have the opportunity to see their clients from the perspective of a variety of roles they assume. In the opening case,

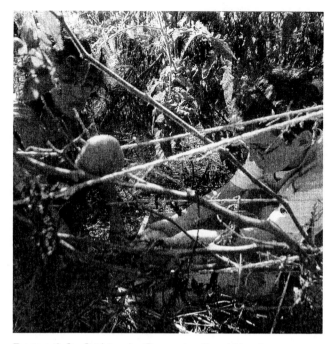

FIGURE 6.3   Bridging the Occupation-Based Meaning

the occupational therapist acknowledges his friend's changed values and beliefs in what is meaningful. The understanding comes from exploration of occupation-based meanings. The following examples illustrate the high value that therapists place on understanding the individual in the community through their life occupations and on relating to those concerns in interactions.

Therapists have the advantage of being objective professionals who can interpret a client's difficulties in measurable ways. "I always give hope and tell clients that they will not always feel this way," says Kathy Hanlon. "I might find something related to their 'occupation' that might draw them out if they are withdrawn. I always try to help people look at the hopeful side of things, but not in a patronizing kind of way."

By giving objective feedback to the client, the therapist helps clients realize things they could not previously acknowledge about their ability to function. "I always try to relate what is going on in the session to the bigger picture related to occupation," continues Hanlon. "I try to make what is going on in the session applicable to what is going on outside the session in the person's life. That is the purpose of the session."

LISTENING

There are many examples of engaging and connecting in the therapists' narratives. Listening is essential to these processes. The therapists are highly active in using all of the techniques identified as components of interactive reasoning. Listening serves as a foundation for all the interactions. Therapists, as illustrated in the forthcoming comments, value active listening and use it to inform their interactive reasoning. This involves examining body language, reading verbal and nonverbal cues, and considering latent and manifest content in communications.

"There are examples of what has worked in the past, and that I understand because I have seen them before," says Ellen Cohen Kaplan. "I use a lot of levity. This involves smiling, body language, and what you and they say. Yes, they recognize it."

Kathy Hanlon agrees. "You read nonverbal communication, and that is so important. Everything from facial expression to sitting, for example."

Other cues that therapists listen for are verbal. "Some of the concrete cues, like how they are responding to questions, tell me a lot about whether I have to repeat things," says Thayer McCain. "If I pick up a more passive or resistive behavior, I have to explain more than I would for those who buy into it at first. With others, it is more clear from the beginning that they will buy into it."

UNDERSTANDING AND USE OF NARRATIVE/SYMBOLIC

In the chapter opening case study, the occupational therapist tells the story using several symbols and metaphors. (See Critical Case Question 6.4.) His narrative gives voice to what is going on in his own mind as the evening unfolds. As a therapist, he can use his story along with the client's to build a portrayal of the future as a means toward establishing empathy as well as validating each experience.

The use of narrative and the symbolic is an extension of understanding the culture of the individual and community. By gaining meaning through use of symbols, the therapist is better able to bridge the cultural worlds of practitioner, client, and family. In the following comment, a community-based occupational therapist captures the use of the narrative and symbolic in what he calls "felt sense."

FELT SENSE

"Felt sense is sensing the way the client can or wants to relate about the pain or the issue," says Thayer McCain. "For instance, in one case, during the first phone call, I gave a woman a hard time; there was something that made me joke with her from the beginning. As it turns out, the woman was blind and had very serious problems. But it worked out fine. Part of [being successful] is having faith, a little faith to act upon this felt sense and awareness, and trying not to be too cognitive. I throw something out and see if it resonates. If it does not, then I change my direction.

"In a way, it is like teaching my kids to drive: They can do some maneuvers in the parking lot, and when I get them out on the road, they cannot do them. There are so many things happening at once that they go too fast or too slow. They lack the experience, such as the feeling of backing up the car, that once you have done it, you know what it is. When starting out as a therapist, I could not trust the felt sense. Everything had to be conscious. Part of it is not knowing what you do not know as a new therapist. You know more than you think you do and less than you think. If I think about going in and being the only person [as in a home setting], I get very caught up in what I have to do. Working with a team allows you to be 'on' and 'off,' like in supervision when you can watch, listen, be 'off' and 'on.'"

BACK TO CARLOS

The future of occupational therapy lies in therapists' going to where the client is—therefore, the community. Carlos illustrates the evolving of community occupational therapy to the extent that he has become the teacher, the driver of therapy. Occupational therapists must take their cues from the clients, which is best achieved in the communities in which they live.

SUMMARY

This chapter presented the themes and techniques of interactive reasoning. The therapists' conscious use of themselves as a tool is essential. The narrative suggests the importance of therapist self-understanding and exposure to a variety of cultures.

REFLECTIVE QUESTIONS

- The ability to examine countertransference reactions is an art and can be practiced. Consider the scenarios described in this chapter. What reactions do you have?
- Go back to the scenarios described in this chapter and other chapters. Who and which situations "push your buttons," and why? What patterns can you identify?
- Think about your life history and experiences. Can you identify patterns in your exposure to various cultures?
- Make a list of cultural perspectives where you lack exposure. What opportunities exist for you to learn more about these cultures and to heighten your sensitivity, for example, visit a neighborhood, trying a new recipe or restaurant?
- All therapists can benefit from support as well as the opportunity to safely and confidentially explore and possibly change aspects of themselves that interfere with forming therapeutic relationships in their work. Who are these individuals in your educational program, supervisory staff, or community? Are there concerns you should bring to a counselor, therapist, or spiritual leader outside of your work or school environment?

INFORMATION CHECKPOINTS

6.1. MULTIPLE NARRATIVES

Multiple narratives or stories exist in the culture of community. These perspectives include the

- therapist
- client or student

- program
- employer or company
- community

6.2. EMPATHIC CONNECTIONS

Empathic connections require the ability to set aside your own agenda to listen to and validate the other person's perspective.

6.3. METACOGNITIVE PROCESS

An example of a metacognitive process: Frame it and stay in the moment (Ellen Cohen Kaplan).

6.4. OPEN-ENDED QUESTIONS

The therapist has a real sense of the client and what the person is going through. The therapist sees the person as a real person and not a category. The therapist is asking open-ended questions or making statements like, "I think this may be a place where you are stuck," not, "This is your problem." The therapist is always feeding the information back to the client (Kathy Hanlon).

CRITICAL CASE QUESTIONS

6.1. Identify the various players in the chapter opening case study. Imagine their stories. What might a narrative be from each of the perspectives?

6.2. Upon what basis is Mike making decisions about his interactions with Carlos?

6.3. What are Mike's dilemmas as he struggles with sorting out his own story and needs from Carlos' situation?

6.4. In the chapter opening case study, "motorcycle" becomes a metaphor. What does it mean to you in the story? Can you identify other symbolism in the story and describe it?

KEY TERMS

BRIDGING

Facilitating understanding of occupation-based meanings by exploring the relationship between real situations that occur outside the therapist-client relationship and experiences with the therapist or other clients.

RESISTANCE

Actions that are not necessarily conscious but stand in the way of achieving a goal. The resistance is usually based in an intrapsychic conflict and a needed defense at the moment.

VALIDATE

To demonstrate through words or actions that the other person's concern is understood and accepted.

THE PRACTICE POPULATIONS

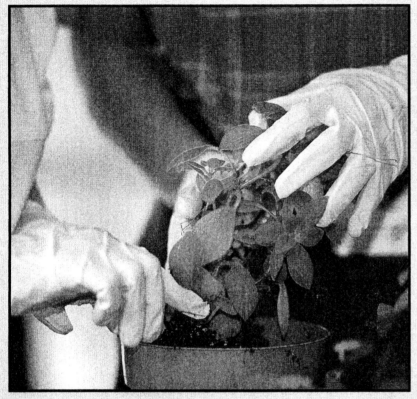

The Power Alliance: An Interactive Reasoning Approach to the Practitioner-Client Relationship

*P*art III discusses the populations that occupational therapists regularly encounter. Although not exhaustive, the sample represents life span issues and the clinical conditions prevalent in an occupational therapist's practice.

Chapter 7 is concerned with children and their families. The situations presented give a range of perspectives from interacting with perceptions of the child with a disability to parents. Following a developmental sequence, chapter 8 presents concerns of the adult. Here the reader will

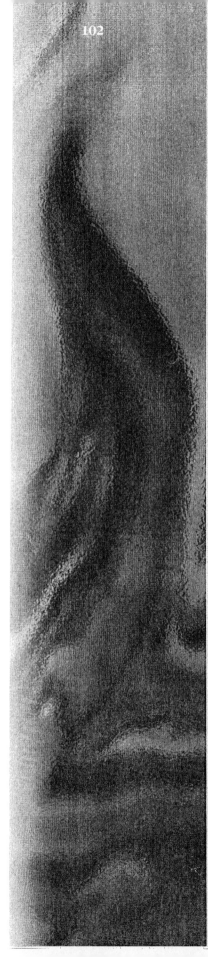

find a wide range of interactive situations. Part III concludes with chapter 9 with the occupational performance concerns of the older adult. We find therapists increasingly working with an older and older population. The caregiver is given special attention in this chapter. Whether in the home or institutional setting, the caregiver is often central to the practitioner's therapeutic role with an individual who is severely disabled or technology dependent.

CHILDREN AND THEIR FAMILIES

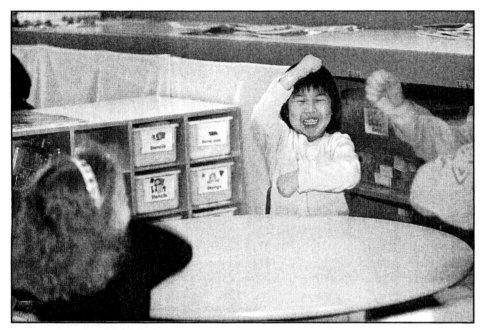

FIGURE 7.1   Building Success through Meaningful and Well-Matched Occupations

SIXTEEN AND SEVERELY ANOREXIC
By Mary Barnes
(January 12, 2000)

*H*eather, 16, is hospitalized for severe anorexia. After several months of successful treatment, she is now gaining and maintaining weight, with close nursing supervision of her meal plan and after coordinating and consulting with a dietitian. Formerly very tearful and subject to extreme mood swings, Heather now either shows no emotion or is momentarily upbeat. She consistently has responded positively to one-on-one or group occupational therapy, during which she becomes involved in activities she finds meaningful. Heather finds soothing activities such as arts and crafts, cleaning the occupational therapy workshop space, and organizing/ordering supplies as part of a vocational group. She also seems calmed by one-on-one sessions with the occupational therapist. Together, they read her journal entries and discuss the meaning of her words and actions in greater detail.

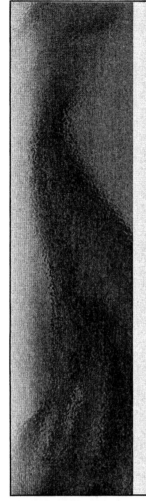

On a trip to the local library with the occupational therapist, Heather checks out a book that details a young woman's personal account of her struggle with eating disorders and her journey to recovery. Later, during a community outing to buy cooking supplies, Heather discloses that she feels she has no coping skills other than her eating-disordered behaviors and that she is angry with her family for being unsupportive. She says they blame her for her eating disorder and for her inability to live at home. In reply, the occupational therapist asks Heather if she can tell her the exact words that her family said to her. The therapist wants to try to assess together whether the words had become distorted by Heather's self-perceptions. Heather replies adamantly that she has been told that her situation is all her fault and that she is starving herself for attention.

Over the weekend, Heather hides food and starts exercising furiously. She loses two pounds and faces the consequence of being restricted to the unit. The psychiatrist and psychologist both confront Heather about her eating behavior and attempts to exercise in secret. Heather responds by shutting down. She agrees to attend her occupational therapy group sessions, but she is quiet and withdrawn. Following the session, the occupational therapist approaches her in private and apologizes for not hearing her cry for help. Heather starts crying and acknowledges the occupational therapist's observation that they need to work at communicating more directly and clearly, saying that she was trying to "hint" that she needed help. The occupational therapist promises to read the book that Heather read on a woman's struggle with eating disorders, and Heather promises to resume her journal writing. The following week, another one of Heather's therapists remarks that Heather has brought her journal to therapy and has begun to open up. She asks Heather if it would be helpful for Heather and the therapist to start meeting with the occupational therapist to work on Heather's issues.

OVERVIEW

Chapter 5 presented therapists' perspectives on working with children and families in the schools. This chapter considers the unique aspects of working with children as a developmental age group in the broader context of the family.

Many populations of children are seen by occupational therapists. (See Information Checkpoint 7.1.) These children have problems that range from acute trauma to concerns related to developmental adjustment. The problems may have a severe or limited impact on occupational performance or component skills and illuminate the themes and techniques of interactive reasoning.

ACTIVE PARTICIPATION AND COLLABORATION

In working with children, family support is essential. As Case-Smith (1997) reported in her study of school-based practice, "the role of family was mentioned in almost every story of success and every story of frustration. When students were successful, the parents were described to be part of the team" (p. 149). In the chapter opening case study, we see how central the family is in the client's system of thinking and to her self-esteem. (See Critical Case Questions 7.1 and 7.2.)

CULTURAL SENSITIVITY TO FAMILY

The therapist needs to take an active role in understanding the family culture. According to Lawlor and Mattingly (1998), "difficulties intensify when there are substantial cultural or socioeconomic gulfs between practitioners and families, for here mistrust and confusion can abound about the roles expected of each. Even the notion of what constitutes 'family' comes into question" (p. 261).

Medhurst and Ryan's (1996a, 1996b) study of the child with a degenerative condition also supports the importance of understanding the family's needs. They propose that "telling the story" of the child and the family's needs to the social service manager helps to clarify underlying meanings in events that are unfolding. The themes relate to solving practical problems: time, adjustment periods, and multiple interpretations of the same story by family members with differing roles. In the following narratives, these same concerns are expressed.

The therapists who were interviewed conceptualized their approaches in a number of ways, including using the following themes: the family system, the use of empowerment, the parent as observer, family play, and parental development.

THE FAMILY SYSTEM

"In pediatrics, you are always working with the family system!" says Sharon Ray, OTR/L, of the Boston School of Occupational Therapy at Tufts University in

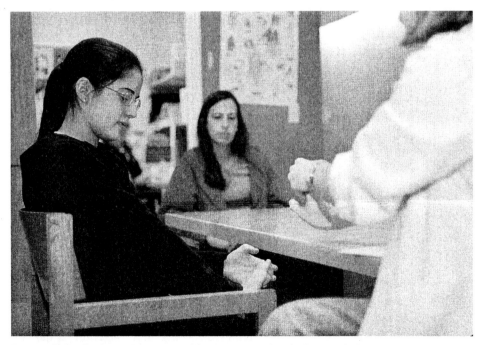

FIGURE 7.2   Exploring, Listening, and Understanding Family-Centered Motives

Medford. "This takes place at the legal level, in regards to what you need to provide according to the law, as well as at the clinical level. The family is responsible for the child's progress. That is especially true when you work with caregivers of the young child. The therapist needs to ask who the players are in the family, because it is not always obvious; for example, in one family, the decision maker might be the grandmother." (See Information Checkpoint 7.2.)

"By couching," says Ray, "you can involve the parent and take the focus away from the problem. It may be too threatening to talk directly about the problem, but talk around the issue, and then get the players involved. Look at how each person is using nonverbal cues. The goal is to work with the family as a team. You want them to know you care about the parent as well as the child." In couching, the therapist is talking about the concerns in a language and manner that is palatable to the parent.

LEARNING TO EMPOWER

During rapport building, the therapist validates the family's concerns, says Ray. "The therapist makes an initial plan and follows the lead of the caregiver and the family. It is important to empower parents to measure a child's progress so that you become a team player, and teach them to recognize what is going on, for example, by giving them markers or what to look for, such as being able to identify motor control problems in cerebral palsy."

In pediatrics, it is not only the child who is the focus of therapeutic intervention but also the family dynamic. In setting therapeutic goals, therapists try to give the family the tools with which to identify and fix problems in the family as they come up. "I would aim to help educate and to help the family make informed decisions at points of progress," says Sharon Ray. "For example, the therapist gives reasons why the child is not progressing and continually relates the conversation back to the caregiver's perspective. What I do with parents is fifty percent listening and fifty percent educating."

To reach parents, therapists must be able to communicate effectively and to meet the parents at their level. "With the parent, the key is getting them involved," says Laura Snell, OTR/L, of the Bay Cove Early Intervention Center in Dorchester. "When parents become involved, they 'get it' and start coming up with their own ideas. That is when the connection is made."

"Empower the parents by educating them," says Ray, "by understanding the reasons for their concerns and by guiding them to find things to look for that would further the therapeutic goals. Empower parents no matter who they are; then you are building trust. Do not use jargon unless the family needs it."

PARENT AS OBSERVER

The therapist often looks to the parent to provide carryover following therapy when the therapist cannot be present. "The elements of interactive reasoning really depend on what I feel the parent can handle at the time, especially in the clinic when we are working on lots of different areas," says Katie McCarthy, OTR/L, of Occupational Therapy Associates in Watertown. "The question is whether I can ask the parents to carry over specific things at home. If I feel they are overwhelmed, then I will suggest only one thing or ask for one idea from the parents to replicate something we have been working on in the clinic. If the family is receptive to ideas, then I would suggest activities that are organizing or enabling the child to focus on tasks. I take my cues from the parents. I adapt my interactions on the basis of the parent's receptivity. If the parents are not ready for suggestions, I just talk about the sessions and the types of things that have worked in the child's school setting and what has worked at home."

Debbie Caruso, OTR/L, of the Brookline Public Schools, also finds that in optimal situations, the family applies the results of treatment in the home setting. But she notes that this will not happen automatically. The therapist must take the time to educate the family members in how to apply in the home the principles they learn in therapy. "When you don't have time with the families for carry-through, it is very frustrating," she says. "Also, it is very helpful for the opportunity to work with siblings. They can learn how to play with their sibling who has a problem. For example, a sibling can learn that it is not helpful to tickle a brother or sister with sensory integration issues because it upsets them."

ENGAGING/CONNECTING AND CREATING A HOLDING ENVIRONMENT

To connect with the child or family, therapists adapt their behavior so that a good match occurs. In the following examples we learn what therapists think about as they engage, connect, and create a holding environment. Therapists describe situations in which they are successful in making the connections.

The adaptations therapists devise require analysis of the neuro-sensory-motor, cognitive, and psychosocial needs of the child and demands of the activity. In the chapter opening case study, the therapist reports that Heather appears soothed by activities such as arts and crafts, cleaning the occupational therapy

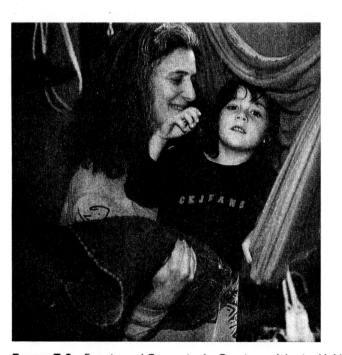

FIGURE 7.3   Engaging and Connecting by Creating an Adaptive Holding Environment

workshop space, and organizing/ordering supplies as part of a vocational group. She also reports observations of other calming sessions, where in a one-on-one interaction the relationship and activity were meaningful to the young adult. (See Critical Case Question 7.3.) In another situation, the therapist decides to lower her voice and modify body movements so as not to further excite a hyperaroused child.

Therapists move between interactive reasoning and procedural reasoning. One type of reasoning informs the other. To create the holding environment and connecting relationship, the therapist must analyze the meaning of the activity as well as adjust the task and interaction so that the child feels validated and a connection is made.

INTERPRETING FAMILY DYNAMICS

"You need to build rapport, in order to gain trust and to gather information," says Sharon Ray. "Who is the decision maker? How can you build trust with the family so that they are comfortable making disclosures? It is important to understand cultural aspects in order to develop openness and trust.

"Having clear guidelines is very important," continues Ray. "Read the children's cues. For the disturbed child, the child with a severe behavioral disorder, having clear guidelines is especially important. The other thing I look at is alternatives, giving a place for connection. This requires that the therapist make a shift, go with the person, and not assign blame."

Mary Barnes conceptualizes the challenge in terms of the theory behind developmental issues. "What is developmentally appropriate and acceptable, as well as effective within the hospital context?" she asks. "This involves creating a holding environment through use of such techniques as containment, feedback, redirecting, and cues, which are part of the object relations frame of reference. Therapists in a group setting should always consider the group as a whole from the perspective of how to keep the member in check in the group, for example, giggling and laughing. An ideal group would need me less and would be more like a 'mature' group." Using an object relations frame of reference, therapists through their actions substitute for the child's diminished ego functioning and impaired early attachments.

FAMILY PLAY

Family play is important to the child's development and to the bonding of the group as a cohesive, supportive unit. Nancy Keebler, a graduate student at Tufts University, Boston School of Occupational Therapy in Medford, Massachusetts, explains family play as a context for intervention. She observes the following. A therapist's knowledge of how a family plays together informs the treatment process. Where, when, and how a family plays together indicates what the family values. It is a piece of how a family spends time together, specifically of what the family views as recreation. It is a part of the family routine. Sometimes play is segregated from routine, such as doing laundry without the children; sometimes it is integrated, as in cooking and doing dishes, in which children are incorporated into the routine. Cultures differ as to how they interpret this. Interventions that the occupational therapist uses need to fit in with the family's routine. Interventions can use play as a therapeutic modality to develop play skills, for example, visual-motor skills, head control, and tracking. Therapists should facilitate playfulness in creating a safe environment and in communicating to the child that he or she is in control. Therapists can propose patterns of play that fit into the family context as well as to the child's level of development. The therapist can suggest where this could take place in the family's environment, when, and with what types of materials.

Whether the therapist uses play or some other modality with the family, the challenge is to address therapeutic goals for the child and the family. "If things are going right, the other person's priorities and interests are involved in what we are doing, and he or she is excited," says Marion Sitomer, OTR/L, of the Anne Sullivan Center Early Intervention Program in Lowell. "Depending on the age of the child, this excitement could be indicated by a facial expression and affect or a willingness to cooperate. That can be true even for an infant. Treatment is a cooperative effort, and infants are expressing their own ideas of the activity. Babies are wired to learn through fun and play."

PARENTAL DEVELOPMENT

"With the parent and the other professionals, it is very much the same if the therapy process is free-flowing. Therapy is a family service, so if things are going well for the child, parental interaction is just as crucial. The therapist needs to determine where the parent is in his or her development as a parent and where the parent is in meeting his or her child's needs. It is sort of the same for the professional, particularly in early intervention, which is very transdisciplinary. If the professionals do not work together, therapy will not be effective. We all have to learn from each other and do things to complement each other. If things are going right, I am learning, too. I am satisfied. Knowing that there is a connection is the biggest part of it." Therapists all seem to agree that parental involvement is key because early intervention is a systematic attempt to foster the development of the atypical child from the onset. The constituted family and parents learn interactive reasoning from the therapists in the case of successful interventions.

This therapeutic process is an expression of the multitrack mind (Fleming), notes Sitomer. "You are picking up cues from at least two people, parent and child, for example. You are looking for flow by engaging the person, motivating him or her, and thinking about the sensory systems of the child. You may be looking at overload or overarousal or to see if the child's fatigue is distracting or overloading. The therapy process is seeing the learning styles of the child and parent, in terms of responsiveness, irritability, and so forth. In the moment, I am not conscious of it until I get a signal that I must pay attention to one of those things."

ROLE OF INTUITION

"For example," Sitomer continues, "if I am trying to keep the focus on the child and the parent needs to talk about an unrelated matter, I have to take a moment to think about whether I should allow her to say what is on her mind or focus on the child. Should I deal with the parent's issue? If the child is losing interest, why? If the child is fatiguing, why? All of these things are going on at the same time below the surface, and when something erupts, then I must pay attention. It is the intuitive piece that fits all the theory — systems theory, group dynamics, etc.—together. The thing that complicates this is that all [the family members] are at a different developmental level. It can be difficult to identify the unifying focus of therapy. That is where you can learn a tremendous amount from others on the team."

Katie McCarthy finds that working in the home is the most effective therapeutic environment because it is holistic. "This can happen in early intervention," she says. "You have all the players immediately present in the home. When you are working with a family or in the clinic and the family members are able to use the information you have given them, it is such a dynamic interaction. The family is feeling empowered. At the start of therapy, parents are usually in a state of confusion and do not know what to do. As they understand the child more, especially how the child's sensory system has been part of the family system, they begin to understand some strategies that they can use to adapt to the situation. In contrast, the family members may not be present in the clinic, so the child is seen in isolation. In the school environment where I work, I do not have all the players; some of the players are frequently absent. However, when therapy is working in the school setting, the teacher is able to carry over adaptations into the classroom. Teachers take the ball and run. With the child, when therapy is working, it is 'magical.' [Children] want to grow."

EXPLORING AND INTERPRETING MOTIVES AS WELL AS OCCUPATION BASED MEANINGS

Self-esteem is central to psychosocial functioning of the child as well as the family. Case-Smith (1997) in her study of narratives of school-based practitioners found that sense of self and self-esteem were important goals in occupational therapy. She observed that therapists reported self-esteem to be an important, if not the most important, outcome of successful intervention.

The following narratives illustrate therapists' use of occupation, meanings, and actions in their interactive reasoning. Special attention is given to adapting the activity and to building success and self-esteem for both the child and the family.

"Having been trained in the sensory integration area, I rely heavily on the child-directed approach," says Katie McCarthy. "I am concerned with what these children are telling me by how they are handling their environment in multiple settings. How can they lead me to the type of sensory input they need? With the child, you can't say, 'Let's do this, based on the parent.' You have to see the child first. The concepts I use from the sensory integration literature are the child-directed and therapist-guided approaches."

"When working with children, you have to suspend your judgement," says Laura Snell, OTR/L, of the Bay Cove Early Intervention Center in Dorchester. "The focus is on how you can help the young client change his behavior even when you will not be there, for example, when he is sledding or on a swing. What can be done when the child is screaming in the park? How can he be calmed, for example, using oral motor input [things to chew] and movement—such as keeping the stroller moving? If he has sensory integration problems, what kinds of things will give him an outlet? In one situation, the client's mother is very involved. I have spent time teaching her how to think in a sensory framework.

Recently, she volunteered that her son likes to wear a tight cap when he eats. This is an example of a mother's taking the ball and running with it."

LISTENING

Listening involves both verbal and nonverbal components. The therapist studies the child and family from multiple systems such as the social, neurological, and cognitive. In the chapter opening case study, the therapist uses missed cues to listen more thoroughly to the teenager's cry for help. The following descriptions illustrate how therapists listen when working with children and parents.

"The elements of reasoning can be subtle," says Laura Snell. "Reality is not always the way it is told to you. For example, parents may start talking about the [family members'] relationship with the father. I try to reflect and listen actively. What is theory telling me? It tells me not to pass judgement and not to be personally involved in the conversation. I am trying to help the parents get at what they are feeling and reflect what they are saying to help them help themselves, to help the parents see that there are options without giving them the answers."

Often, therapists have to work at picking up a family's cues. "Even if the child is having a good time with what I am doing, if I am not getting feedback from the child, I am not picking up the cues," says Marion Sitomer. "It has to flow both ways. With issues related to pervasive developmental disabilities (PDD), it is really hard to detect the cues. With the kids who cannot even make eye contact, I have to really work hard. The same applies to parents. I have to know when to pick up with the parent. It is very challenging sometimes."

UNDERSTANDING AND USE OF NARRATIVE/SYMBOLIC

The value of understanding the symbolic elements in communication and activities comes up in therapists' responses and choices. The chapter opening case study presents opportunities for symbolic analysis. (See Critical Case Question 7.4.) Therapists listen to the child and family narratives within a developmental context to interpret and understand meanings.

"You must work with the mind-body connection in interactive reasoning," says Mary Barnes. "That is why with adolescents I am careful about my appearance. The mind-body connection guides how quickly I use facial expressions, the content of my language."

BACK TO HEATHER

Being honest in the way one expresses and conducts oneself as a therapist is difficult, even for the experienced therapist. However, as we see in the chapter opening case study, despite such difficulty the payoff can be rewarding. The therapist apologizes for not heeding Heather's cry for help. The therapist's frank and courageous admittance of a mistake is the ultimate interactive reasoning, where the therapist is connecting at the most revealing level, and by so doing the therapist is showing she is willing to go the extra mile to work with the client.

SUMMARY

In this chapter on interactive reasoning, the family is an integral part of considering the child and young adult. All the themes and techniques as well as supporting narratives from the therapist's interview support a family-centered approach rather than expert driven care. Adaptation is essential to the therapist's reasoning and action with children and young adults. Rather than create dependency on the therapist, the aim is to empower the child and family through appropriate resources and experiences.

REFLECTIVE QUESTIONS

- Family systems and cultures are central to interactive reasoning about the child. Think about your own family system and culture. What was your experience, and how does it affect your values and expectations of others?
- How might your values about family and the role of children come into conflict with other groups in your work as an occupational therapist?
- What influences might your family-oriented perspectives have on your interactive reasoning and actions as a therapist? When might these attitudes be effective or ineffective?
- Parenting experiences are significant to a therapist's interactive reasoning. Like other health professionals, many occupational therapists have a family member or person close to them who has been chronically ill or has a disability. Reflect upon your own background. Identify how your emotional needs that result from your relationships with others might be displaced in a therapeutic setting. Describe both positive and negative consequences.

INFORMATION CHECKPOINTS

7.1. CHILDREN

Occupational therapists work with children who have a variety of problems. A sample list of the problems include children who are medically fragile and technology dependent, children and teens with HIV/AIDS, children who are deaf or hearing impaired or have low vision, teens with mental health and substance abuse problems, children with sensory-integrative dysfunction, young adults with traumatic brain injury, children with developmental disabilities, and children with chronic, degenerative conditions.

7.2. FAMILY-CENTERED CARE

In family-centered care, "perspectives of both parties should be altered as they gain and consider new information brought about through a collaborative process" (Lawlor & Mattingly, 1998, p. 260).

CRITICAL CASE QUESTIONS

7.1. Imagine you are Heather, the 16-year-old girl hospitalized because of anorexia. Tell the story of your life. What is it like to be with your parents at mealtime? What do they expect of you?

7.2. Imagine you are the father or mother of Heather. Tell the story of your life. What was it like for you as a child? What is it like to be with your daughter at mealtime?

7.3. Imagine you are the occupational therapist responsible for treating Heather. Where do you believe you made an error in your attempts to connect with Heather? Based upon the narratives and stories you constructed in questions 7.1 and 7.2, how do you think Heather perceived your comments, and why?

7.4. As stated in the chapter opening case study, Heather appears soothed by activities such as arts and crafts, cleaning the occupational therapy workshop space and organizing/ordering supplies as part of a vocational group. She also appears calmed by one-on-one sessions with the occupational therapist during which they read her journal entries and discuss the meaning of her words and actions in greater detail. What meaning and themes possibly exist in these activities? What relationship do you see between Heather's response to the activities, her reaction in the one-on-one sessions with the occupational therapist, and the therapist's intervention?

KEY TERMS

CHILD-DIRECTED APPROACH

An approach that is concerned with what the child is telling the therapist by how the child is handling his or her environment in multiple settings (Katie McCarthy).

FAMILY-CENTERED CARE

Intervention shaped by the family rather than by the professionals alone as the experts.

FAMILY SYSTEM

The composite of people deeply or peripherally involved in a child's life that may include biologic or nonbiologically related parents, grandparents, great grandparents, siblings, and extended family members such as aunts, uncles, and cousins as well as caregivers, babysitters, and neighbors. Children may have more than one family system as a result of remarriage, change of partners, adoption, divorce, and so forth. The culture of each system may vary in terms of religion, ethnicity, sexual orientation, etc.

MIDDLE- AND LATER-AGED ADULTS, FRIENDS, FAMILY, AND PARTNERS

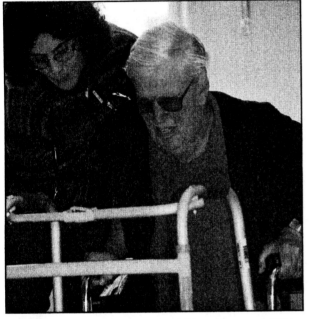

FIGURE 8.1 Collaboration through Mental Imagery in Talking the Task

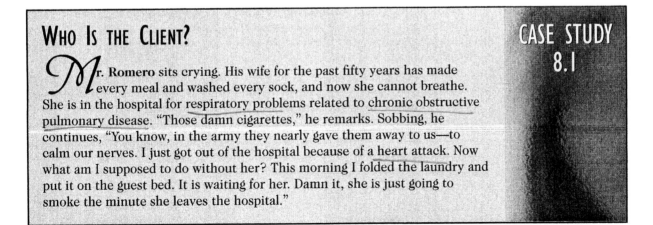

WHO IS THE CLIENT?

*M*r. Romero sits crying. His wife for the past fifty years has made every meal and washed every sock, and now she cannot breathe. She is in the hospital for respiratory problems related to chronic obstructive pulmonary disease. "Those damn cigarettes," he remarks. Sobbing, he continues, "You know, in the army they nearly gave them away to us—to calm our nerves. I just got out of the hospital because of a heart attack. Now what am I supposed to do without her? This morning I folded the laundry and put it on the guest bed. It is waiting for her. Damn it, she is just going to smoke the minute she leaves the hospital."

OVERVIEW

*T*his chapter focuses on middle- and later-aged adult populations. Functional problems common to this group typically result from stroke, spinal cord injury, chronic pain, cardiopulmonary conditions, and musculo-orthopedic conditions, including hand and sports injuries.

Sensitivity to role changes and the client's intimate relationships, such as those with friends and partners, should be given special attention in interactive reasoning. As one can see in the chapter opening case study, concerns are multiple and interrelated. (See Critical Case Question 8.1.) Insufficient attention is presented in the literature to the developmental and family needs of occupational therapy with the middle- and later-aged adult.

The impact of institutional environments and community settings is evident in earlier therapist representations of interactive reasoning with adults. The separation of the developmental needs from the context of intervention is artificial. Therapists employ similar strategies with adults in a variety of places, such as the outpatient clinic, community program, and hospital. The following descriptions show the breadth and depth of their interactive reasoning and use of a variety of strategies.

ACTIVE PARTICIPATION AND COLLABORATION

Drawing upon the existential roots of the profession, occupational therapists engage clients through understanding the world of their clients. As Crepeau (1991) wisely explains, "Because occupational therapists must 'do with' for treatment to be successful, their achievement of intersubjective understanding is critical" (p. 1019). (See Critical Case Questions 8.2 and 8.3.) Therapists describe how they use their understanding of the clients' worlds to understand and intervene. The themes of their interactions with clients include such categories as returning control, being mindful, the role of intuition, the bottom line, the importance of family, and reading cues.

Deborah Rochman, OTR/L, of the Tufts University, Boston School of Occupational Therapy, and Dental School, uses a self-management paradigm that is designed to help the person feel in control of his or her pain. "All interventions are geared toward helping the person take control over his or her life," she says. "I have seen people pull their life together." Collaborating with and actively listening to what the patient is saying are essential to dealing with chronic pain, says Rochman. "It is incredible to be able to tune in and really see how pain has affected the person. Collaboration is essential to finding creative ways to get through the day. It is all about problem solving. It is usually the patients who come up with the ideas. They think of things, we discuss them, and usually an idea gets unfolded. Then they try it, and it works."

RETURNING CONTROL

Even in a hospital setting, it is possible to let people take control of their pain, note occupational therapists. "I try to acknowledge that being in a hospital bed is very disempowering. But if I view it as part of the patients' recovery, I become a part of their support system. My ideal is to support their dignity. As a therapist, I found the hardest thing of being in a hospital is watching people being stripped of their control. This is especially true with chronic pain patients. I make resources available, provide things that people can find interest in and can learn from, and help patients start to take control of their pain. I look at how the hospital setting could be more conducive to learning." Part of taking control of pain is the client's learning to be in charge of his or her environment. For example, by making decisions about such things as their daily routines, clients can enhance feelings of well-being.

The occupational therapist can offer clients a plan of action, even if it is simply a new way of viewing something, as a way to gain control. "The best interactive reasoning occurs when patients are motivated, they are progressing and they are really interacting," says Kim Quamme, OTR/L, of the Beth Israel Deaconess Medical Center in Boston. "I'm doing hands-on things and talking them through the therapy process, and hopefully they can participate. If the family are there, they would be involved in what the plan is. I explain the plan, and get the patient to buy into it and commit to something he or she wants to accomplish."

ENGAGING/CONNECTING AND CREATING A HOLDING ENVIRONMENT

Therapists describe their reasoning in terms of engaging, connecting, and establishing rapport with the client. They need to address two main questions: First, how can I get to know this individual? Second, how can I relate to this person in a way he or she understands and that is meaningful for him or her?

"One thing that makes a difference to my being ready to be that person's therapist is being 'present,'" says Janet Curran Brooks, OTR/L, of the Boston School of Occupational Therapy at Tufts University. "I have to 'hang up' whatever is going on personally and professionally, even things that relate to the patient but have nothing to do with the immediate interaction. (See Information Checkpoint 8.1.) This requires a lot of breathing! Many people now call it 'mindfulness.' In order for the session to go well, it has to happen. I do not think you can connect with everyone, but if there is a chance, it should happen, because the patient may not be able to do it."

BEING MINDFUL

Acting mindful yields results, even if not at first, notes Curran Brooks. "One patient in acute care was so angry that she beat me with a reacher! At the SNF [skilled nursing facility] she became civil and cooperated, and then at home, she was pleasant and interactive. She even baked bread before I got there and was cooperative. This type of behavior relates to control, specifically to control of bodily functions, eating slowly, deciding whether or not to have a bowel movement, etc."

Connecting with the client requires looking beyond the client's role as a client. "You are picking up on a million things," continues Curran Brooks. "How do you know what you are doing? Through connecting and recognizing that I have to let the patients be my guide. One time, I visited a patient who was very ill at her home. I walk into her apartment, and the lights are dim. I don't know what is going on. In fact, the patient is in bed, and all of the members of her church are surrounding her. I honestly did not see them until I got close to the patient. I literally blocked out every other distraction except for what was happening with the patient. I had to learn this by doing it."

The difficulty is in getting the person engaged with you, says Deborah Rochman. "That is the big challenge. Establishing rapport is the very first thing you need to do. When it is happening, patients feel safe, know you are listening and that you care about them. The real work is getting the person to make changes. If I act discouraged, because getting patients to change their behavior is really hard, patients will resist my efforts, and not cooperate. So I present a positive and hopeful perspective. A therapist has to. This is common sense."

THE ROLE OF INTUITION

Repeatedly, therapists say that when they use the interactive approach with clients, especially with clients who are in pain, they become involved personally in a way that is difficult to put into words. "I think that interactive reasoning probably is in part intuition," says Michael Nardone, OTR/L, of the University of Hartford. "I think about the therapeutic relationship and the use of touch. People have told me that therapists have a 'soft touch' with burn patients. This makes me think about Ann Mosey [occupational therapy theorist], in terms of performing the art of practice and human interaction. I always feel I am getting something from the patients. Even though it sounds weird, I really feel that there is an energy connection, and I do not think it is only from therapeutic touching."

Nardone had one patient, who was Vietnamese, with whom he closely connected. "I was really interested in this man. We really had fun. He left the hospital a happy man." Nardone attributes some of his success at connecting with patients to his parochial school background, which he describes as "experiencing the joy of giving in a safe community."

THE BOTTOM LINE

"What I like about OT is that every person's situation is always different," says Rebecca Reynolds, OTR/L, of the Concord Seabury School and Animals As Intermediaries. "There is no 'A, B, C' format. What you do depends upon how ready the person is and where the team is. If it is a complex medical situation, then it is pretty straightforward. Regardless, being able to assess safety is always the first part of working with someone. This involves grading the task so that the person knows it is achievable. It relates to how hard I push the person. You have to go by instinct and know when to convince someone that he or she has given up."

Therapists who work with people in chronic pain must be attuned to the psychosocial concerns of clients, or else they cannot connect or interact with them effectively. "There is a lot of touching; often patients will hold my hand as I come in or am about to leave, or maintain eye contact," says Sue Brown, OTR/L, of St. Joseph's Hospital in Warwick, Rhode Island. "I think our setting helps facilitate that. A lot of the nurses and OTs introduce us by first names. I start with 'Mr.' or 'Mrs.' and then ask the patients what they prefer. The staff sets the tone. From the minute someone comes in the door, the nurse sees the patient to the room;

therapy comes after that. Another thing we try to do every time before leaving a patient is to ask, 'Is there anything you need, for example, water? To watch TV?' Over time, I believe that helps build rapport."

For some therapists, discussing how they conduct themselves during the interactive process is like naming the streets they drive on to go to work every day—the details are so familiar that they are difficult to recall and can only be described in general. "It is hard, because you don't think of these things [the elements of interactive reasoning]," says Sue Brown. Still, she lists some of the steps involved. "I sit at eye level or below. I always try to explain to the best of their understanding what the activity is and to relate it to their goals. I explain it in relation to the home environment, and I do this in setting up the treatment. I don't know that I could name what theory I use; part of it is intuition and getting to know the patient and his or her history. We have a full range of patients, some functioning at a high level, and some at lower levels. So I adapt my approach to what they would understand."

EXPLORING AND INTERPRETING MOTIVES AS WELL AS OCCUPATION-BASED MEANINGS

To be meaningful and client-motivated, therapeutic interventions are consistent with the client's occupation-based values and sense of self-identity. The therapist achieves this aim through exploration and interpretation of motives through occupation-based meanings. Storytelling, that is, eliciting stories from clients about their past and present, within an occupational context has been suggested as a viable means to this end (Clark, 1993; Price-Lackey & Cashman, 1996). Clark named these practices "occupational storytelling" and "occupational story making" (p. 1074). (See Critical Case Questions 8.4 and 8.5.)

In the chapter opening case study, Mr. Romero is bursting with emotion and stories. He gives the occupational therapist a clear picture of his past and present concerns. It is his future where the plot becomes blurred (". . . what am I supposed to do . . . ?"). The situation is ripe for occupational therapy, as Mr. Romero looks to an uncertain occupational future as retiree, former military man, patient with cardiac disease, and bereaved widower or caretaker for his spouse. The developmental issues for this adult are not atypical. Mr. Romero's self-image and self-esteem are at the heart of his struggle around his occupational roles. The narrative gives the therapist insight about role changes, resulting loss of meaning and sense of competence, and the need to reevaluate goals and consolidate life accomplishments.

Evenson and Roberts (1996) maintain that "interactive reasoning is used when a clinician wants to better understand the client" (p. 31). They identify three important sources of information in their clinical reasoning model for working with individuals who have had a stroke: the client's history, prior level of functioning, and future projections. The family's plan, being associated with the therapist's conditional reasoning, is also important. (See Information Checkpoint 8.2.) These areas of inquiry can be applied to a broad range of middle- and later-aged adult populations.

IMPORTANCE OF FAMILY

The centrality of family is seen in the chapter opening case study. The client is both Mr. Romero and Mrs. Romero. Each of their valued roles will change as a result of the other's capacity to function. In a short interview, Mr. Romero gives the occupational therapist clear indications of his distress. As with Mr. Romero, the following informants' comments illustrate the importance of exploring and interpreting motives and occupation-based meanings through client leads.

"One thing that I learned over time was to allow patients to express themselves and to be comfortable with the silence," says Michael Nardone. "I had to learn not to rush them or push them beyond where they wanted to go. I learned this in Harlem, working with burn patients, and at Sloane Kettering, working with breast cancer patients. I was always learning about something from them. Most of all, I developed a respect for the individual's uniqueness. A person's emotional state is important to me. I would ask the people to tell me about themselves. I would ask them about their life history, work, and family. In Harlem, so many people were wonderful storytellers. In that community, allowing people to tell stories guided me. I allowed myself to joke with them. Having a consistent presence as their therapist, I got to see them go from inpatient to outpatient. The women got to see me as their therapist, which was important. This is true for the burn patients as well as the breast cancer patients. Seeing people scarred and open to the world made me feel protective of them."

LISTENING

Listening involves observation. To be successful listeners, therapists need to put their own issues aside so as to accurately perceive the other person. This may be a big challenge if the therapist has closely identified with the adult client because of similar age, background, or situation. Conversely, it is also a challenge if the client has a frame of reference that is foreign to the therapist. What follows are some of the things therapists report about the way in which listening furthers one's ability to conduct interactive reasoning.

"An important element of interactive reasoning is being accurate perceivers of the patient's progress," says Janet Curran Brooks. "Ask youself, 'Did I put my own issues aside? Can I do an honest evaluation? What is important to know: Is the patient progressing?' When I was beginning, if the patients were not getting better, I assumed it was me. I think there is a middle ground."

Listening involves taking cues from the patient. Deborah Rochman says, "In part, I use standard interview questions. For example, I get patients' previous history of pain treatment. I ask about their typical day. I ask questions related to helping them cope with their pain. I look at the individual's level of understanding and what the person can hear. I use mileposts for myself, such as patients' goals. I struggle between getting the information I need and wanting to go (flow) with the person. Sometimes I do not get enough information and have to go back. It is important for me to listen."

READING CUES

While acknowledging that it is critical to look at a person's functioning, therapists say they look beyond it and that they do so by actively listening to the person. "An element of interactive reasoning is using observational skills to see readiness," says Rebecca Reynolds. "I ask questions such as, 'What piece am I doing? What is the client saying and doing? Is fear a piece of it? Is pain a part of it? What is the underlying motivation?' Always, I try to tease out what I am seeing by using as many cues as possible. What is the framework? What matters? As a starting place, I try to check out assumptions. I consistently consider the spirit of the person, not only the function of the person."

Therapists also stress the importance of reading nonverbal cues. "It is a sense you get from the patient's body language," says Sue Brown. "Patients communicate a lot [nonverbally], and it is a matter of recognizing it. It can take a lot of time, and you may not get to your activity, but in the long run, it may be more beneficial. They are going through a lot of change, and they are experiencing fears and anxiety. There are psychological issues, family concerns, and financial concerns that we may not be addressing. I think it is important just to let patients know you hear them and to take a few moments to reflect back what you are hearing to be sure you are not misunderstanding what is being said. It is funny, but we do not think about these things while we do them. I think validation is a big part of it, that they feel they have an advocate in addition to having someone help them reach their functional goals and plan for discharge. To accomplish this, you have to exercise quick judgement and take into account the person's cognitive and behavioral status. You have to allow people the time to vent, if they can or need to, or at least to talk about their concerns. I believe the patients give you signals. And a lot of therapists miss them! I think you are always observing, analyzing, and reevaluating. You look for what works for the patients. During one of my affiliations, my clinical instructor commented to me about the sense of innocence that I had—the sincere willingness to help. He noted that some people lose that. Trying to maintain a balance is important."

UNDERSTANDING AND USE OF NARRATIVE/SYMBOLIC

Getting to know the whole person is a value held by the occupational therapists interviewed. Understanding the symbolic and the narrative is an important means by which therapists come to understand the person, interact, and intervene. It may be an object in a patient's home or hospital room, for example, that becomes the cue to understanding the person. Institutions can also serve as symbols in a person's life and occupational history.

For Mr. Romero, the army, a powerful symbol, becomes a target of anger. While it represents his courage and masculinity it also symbolizes dependency and loss of faith. It is not unusual for people to displace strong feelings, both positive and negative, onto institutions, such as the government, military, or schools, as well as onto authority figures, such as past teachers. Nonhuman objects also serve to inform the therapist and client about sublimated needs and drives. The following are therapists' descriptions of what they understand through use of the narrative and the symbolic.

"I find it useful to establish rapport with older persons from the start and to get more on a personal level with them," says Laura (Guertin) Impemba, of Healthsouth Braintree Pediatric Rehabilitation at Melrose. "If I am in the room, I might comment about the things that they have in their room. That is how the sessions progress. Rather than focusing on the [therapy] work, they are talking about something that is personal."

LIGHTING THE SPARK

"There are times when motivation isn't apparent, and I don't know what it will take to bring out people's spirit, their curiosity, and to help them reclaim their interest in the world," says Rebecca Reynolds. "What will ignite a person's spark? It may be a moth, the smell of sage. Or it might be taking the dog from the therapy clinic outside. A lot of people who come into rehabilitation settings are very passive. They want someone to 'fix' them and make them better. I try to find what tools the person can use to problem-solve now and in the future. I find that patients who experience chronic pain often lack coping skills. However, there is a tendency to make assumptions about the person that needs to be checked. This is especially true when time is a factor—to be able to see the big picture and to hold that. It helps to have really good coworkers in order to stay open to growing and to humility and being willing to change your course of action."

The information-gathering process that is a part of narrative and the symbolic begins even before the therapist sees the client. "I start by getting information beforehand, to get an idea from the chart of what to expect on the initial visit," says Kim Quamme. "It helps to know what to anticipate. I start with a baseline. I ask, 'What is their cognitive status?' The process is intuitive to some degree. But I try to anticipate problems, and then I do more testing as I become aware of functional problems. If they are uncooperative due to a reason other than personality or not wanting to cooperate, I try to relate to what they want to do or what they did before. I try to elicit some participation, for example, if they have a head injury, by the use of pictures in the room or by use of family members. I think it helps to use information I know about people and their baseline status and to try to focus on something they seem interested in. I just go with what appears of interest during a functional activity. I start with typical activities, such as going to the bathroom, and then I think in terms of the components that are involved in doing the activity. I look to see if they are bumping into the wall, for example, and I ask them if they know they bumped into something. I want to see if the problem is strength, visual neglect, or something else, and then I do further testing. The MOHO [model of human occupation] is useful in looking at the whole person and the settings. It brings everything together. As a new graduate, I always had a form and a plan. Now I am able to gear it more to the individual patient. I walk into the room and think, 'OK, what am I going to do today?' To see what is going on from their, not my, perspective."

BACK TO MR. ROMERO

The occupational therapist listened to Mr. Romero tell his story. By active listening she understood that he was coping with many losses, real and symbolic. There would be changes in his daily routine. His self-concept was suffering because he felt inadequate assuming his wife's chores at home. He had not yet found gratifying ways to spend his time since retirement. He questioned the faith he had in institutions and his own health. Through listening and reflecting back these concerns to Mr. and Mrs. Romero, the occupational therapist was able to help them modify their lifestyles and daily activities. An interactive reasoning approach enabled the therapist to engage the couple to promote their own health and a restored sense of competence.

SUMMARY

Occupational therapists are concerned about clients' feelings of being disempowered and out of control. They attend to these issues in their interactive reasoning. Ultimately, establishing rapport is paramount, as therapists truly want to know the adult as an individual. Therapists' goals are occupation based, and their interactions client or individual centered.

REFLECTIVE QUESTIONS

- How do you act when you feel disempowered and out of control in a situation?
- What triggers the feelings you just described?
- What are ways you have successfully gained a feeling of control and competence when disempowered?
- Are there individuals with whom you identify as an oppressed group? What are the concerns of this group, and do you see similar characteristics in other groups? In what ways is your identification possibly a blind spot in your interactive reasoning as an occupational therapist?
- Identify a few objects in your home that are highly meaningful to you. What do they symbolize? Would their meaning be easily apparent to others or highly disguised unless the person knew you or was familiar with your cultural orientation?

INFORMATION CHECKPOINTS

8.1. BEING PRESENT

"Being present is being ready to be that person's therapist, to be present, to 'hang up' whatever is going on personally and professionally with me" (Janet Curran Brooks).

8.2. SOURCES OF UNDERSTANDING IN INTERACTIVE REASONING (EVENSON & ROBERTS 1996)

- Person's life history
- Person's prior level of function, including occupational roles and environment
- Client's and family's needs, plans, and future projections

[handwritten left margin: —heart disease, b/c heart attack → feel that he will not be able to do all tasks required of him.]

[handwritten left margin: worried about role change. 116]

CRITICAL CASE QUESTIONS

8.1. List all the medical problems you can identify in the case. What are they, and how might they influence a person's functioning?

8.2. Imagine you were Mr. Romero. What is his occupational story as you imagine it from his perspective? *[handwritten: [solider] p.123 feels inadequet in being able to complete his own job]*

8.3. Imagine you were Mrs. Romero. What is her occupational story as you imagine it from her perspective? *[handwritten: [society] I have always done this stuff will I be able to do it again?]*

8.4. Imagine you were the occupational therapist working with Mr. Romero. What occupational story might you make with him?

8.5. Compare the occupational story you would create with Mr. Romero to one you would create with Mrs. Romero and to one you would create with the couple both present. How do the stories compare? *[handwritten: Solider → homemaker → active couple]*

KEY TERMS

INTERNAL FRAME OF REFERENCE

The person's inner world of values, beliefs, and attitudes.

"OCCUPATIONAL STORYTELLING"

The storytelling aspect of clinical reasoning, whereby the person relates stories of childhood occupations that influence who he or she is in the present (Clark, 1993, p. 1047).

"OCCUPATIONAL STORY MAKING"

The story-making aspect of clinical reasoning, whereby the patient and therapist are creating stories of the occupational being that is unknown, evolving, and future-oriented (Clark, 1993, p. 1047).

OLDER ADULTS AND CAREGIVERS

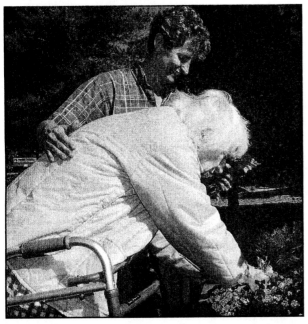

FIGURE 9.1   Active Participation and Collaboration with Just Right Support

SUPPORT GROUP FOR CAREGIVERS

By Scott Trudeau
(June 5, 2000)

I remember leading a patient education group for caregivers of persons with Alzheimer's disease. The group consisted of approximately twelve caregivers, all female, mostly wives (two were daughters) who were all providing day-to-day care for a loved one with a dementing illness. Being an experienced therapist of nearly twelve years of practice, most of which was providing group interventions to adults with mental illness, I was quite confident in my skills to manage this seemingly straightforward session. In fact, I had no idea what I was getting into.

The first noteworthy and unexpected challenges were the facts that I am decidedly male and more than twenty years younger than the youngest group member. As I began to present at the first session, the group was markedly guarded and resistive. I quickly became aware that I was going to have to win their confidence. But how?

It is very important in situations such as this that respect and positive regard are sincerely communicated. It was clear to me, as I emphasized repeatedly to the group, that they were the "experts" at managing persons with dementia at home. I knew very little about the day-to-day challenges they faced; my role in the group was to provide some structure and organization to facilitate each member sharing her own expertise. This began to set the tone for group members to participate.

Another strategy employed early on in this situation was the use of humor. I disclosed with the group some of the times when I had dealt with persons with dementia when something funny had occurred. This served to break the tension but also helped establish my credibility as someone familiar with the trials of dealing with persons with this difficult and debilitating condition.

These initial strategies laid the foundation for a therapeutic relationship between me and the members of the group, which proved invaluable as the sessions progressed. At our final session, the topic to be discussed was home safety. The discussion was active as we critiqued strategies that members had developed to manage everything from access to medications to wandering behavior. As the session was wrapping up, one of the members raised her hand and asked how she could keep her husband from using the snowblower in the road, as she was afraid he might get hit by a plow.

I was blown away! Had she not listened to anything we had discussed? My initial response was to be very critical of her and to demand that she remove the snowblower from her property. However, I drew a deep breath and considered the tone we had set in the group. As such, before I responded, I opened it up for other members to share similar concerns and things they had done to manage similar situations. This proved to be remarkably more therapeutic than my critical tone would have been. As the discussion ensued, it became clear to me that there was much more to the situation than simply providing safety. Here was a woman who had relied on her husband for more than fifty years to shovel the driveway. To some extent reflective of her generation, she was at the same time subservient to and dependent on this man, who now lacked the cognitive capacity to care for her.

The sensitivity and warmth, as well as the shared perspectives from her peers, were incredible to witness. We were able to establish a plan to disable the snowblower, but the sharing and grieving that occurred during this interaction was far more therapeutic than this tangible outcome.

OVERVIEW

*O*ccupational performance problems associated with the older adult are addressed in the therapists' clinical reasoning. The concerns of this population range from those that stem from normal aging to those that result from disease. They may include the older person with depression, dementia, Alzheimer's disease, and chronic obstructive pulmonary disease, for example. Also addressed are the repercussions of aging and the disease processes on the loved ones of the older persons. Caregivers and family members are affected, too.

The special circumstances of the dying client, death and mourning, as well as relationships with caregivers are essential in discussions of interactive reasoning of the occupational therapist who works with the older adult. A strong emphasis on family-centered care is a thread we saw in chapter 7 in the discussion on children. The same focus returns in therapists' discussions and the literature on interactive reasoning with the older adult. The notion of family is extended to more directly include nonrelated caregivers for the elderly population. The older adults of concern in this chapter are also described in earlier chapters that presented interactive reasoning in the inpatient hospital and community setting. Here the unique applications of interactive reasoning with this age group are under consideration.

As one can see in the chapter opening case study, the occupational therapist plays an important role in family education. (See Critical Case Question 9.1.) As with other populations, such as school-based practice, intervention requires that the therapist work within multiple formats with the identified care receiver, the caregivers, or a combination of both. The formats include one-to-one, couples, family, consultation, and group. Although the themes and techniques of interactive reasoning are relevant to all formats, each modality has its unique requirements that call for specialized skills. (See Information Checkpoint 9.1.) The structure of each of the formats calls forth a range of skills and roles on the part of the therapist. (See Information Checkpoints 9.2 and 9.3.) Occupational therapy education at a minimum includes knowledge of the practice of group work and consultation. However, further education is usually required for more than rudimentary work with couples and families or any of the prior formats. In the chapter opening case study, we see the therapist applying a variety of skills and roles in the support group. (See Critical Case Questions 9.2 and 9.3.)

ACTIVE PARTICIPATION AND COLLABORATION

Professional caregiver goals may not always match those of the lay practitioner or family caregiver. Hasselkus (1989) conducted a study of the meaning of *caregiving* in terms of the caregivers for frail older people living in the community. She found that the forms of caregiving activities were determined by these practitioners' judgements regarding the prioritization and attainment of goals. (See Information Checkpoint 9.4.) Further, because of potential perceived differences, the relationship between the professional caregiver and lay caregivers needs careful consideration and discussion (Hasselkus, 1989, 1994). As we will see in therapists' reports, all the players' values and goals directly influence the occupational therapists' interactions and reasoning about interventions with the older adults and caregivers. The themes touched on by the therapists interviewed include eliciting cooperation, making the connection, being true to self, being present, and using observational skills.

As in every therapeutic relationship, communication is key to working with older adults. Special attention needs to be given to the use of metaphors and nonverbal aspects of communication in reasoning about interactions with adults with dementia. Perrin and May (2000) emphasize that metaphors in dementia care help us understand what the person would say if the ability to communicate meaning were present "in this world of figure and shadow and type" (p. 102). They also advise validating the person's feelings as often as possible and keeping a running commentary about what has just happened and is about to occur. The following therapist, an expert in caring for individuals with severe dementia and Alzheimer's disease, describes his experience. He emphasizes, as do Perrin and May (2000), the importance of making eye contact as a basic tool of communication at a primitive level.

"This population requires multiple levels of interactive reasoning," says Scott Trudeau, OTR/L, Edith Nourse Rogers Memorial VAMC, Bedford, Massachusetts, and Tufts University Boston School of Occupational Therapy, Medford, Massachusetts. "You start at the primitive level with people who are severely demented by establishing eye contact. The next level is interaction with the family: What is the family dynamic? Is that coloring their interaction, such as in denying an abusive relationship with the identified patient?"

ELICITING COOPERATION

Interactions with people who are mentally ill can call for creative solutions. "I think the best therapy is when I work with someone who brings questions and ideas to the therapy session," says Dalit Waller, OTR/L, with the Neville Manor Nursing Home, an affiliate of the Cambridge-Somerville Health Alliance. "It involves collaboration, and it takes place in all settings. However, I would say that it is rare. One example of how it happens: I saw a man with schizophrenia who is in his 50s, who has very poor mobility. He was having trouble with night-time toileting. He always came with ideas, and together we arrived at a solution. This was hospital-level rehabilitation. I think the first thing I do is try to get a sense of what the client's concerns are regarding therapy. I try to elicit the person's goals. For example, they say they want to walk. They probably need physical therapy. Then the goal becomes trying to elicit what else matters to them and what they are having trouble with. Sometimes they do not know. So we need to take the time to talk with the person, to take him or her through the task."

In talking with the client, the therapist is analyzing aloud the steps of the activity in the context of the setting as if she were there during the activity. She might say, "Imagine you wake in the middle of the night feeling the urge to urinate. It is dark and you don't know where you are," and so on and so forth. Involving the person at each moment, the therapist goes over the steps of one piece of an activity literally as if she were walking the patient through it.

The therapists' use of interactive reasoning is tempered by the type of client with whom the therapists are working. "Interactive reasoning often entails going with the flow," says Wally VanDyck, OTR/L, with St. Joseph's Hospital, Warwick, Rhode Island. "In head injury, for example, the patient might not know what is going on. In the beginning, that is what might happen until we can introduce structure. We may defer to other qualified individuals to explain the patient's condition. It depends on the patient population. The more I understand who the person is, what has meaning to him or her, and what his or her values are, the more I can incorporate those elements. The driving force is keeping patients focused to maximize our use of time so that they get things accomplished according to what they want."

ENGAGING/CONNECTING AND CREATING A HOLDING ENVIRONMENT

Therapists work very hard at establishing a relationship with the care recipient. How to be in the therapeutic relationship is at the heart of what a therapist thinks about and focuses on. It can be summarized as being real, trying out different interactive styles, and adapting to the person and situation.

In the chapter opening case study, the support group provides a holding environment. As caregivers, the group members are the experts. Because of their lived experience, they are credible witnesses and legitimize issues and remedies. The therapist's role is to facilitate and create an environment whereby the support group thrives and can provide technical expertise and can also act as a resource.

A holding environment is essential to effective care with older individuals with dementia. Perrin and May (2000) strongly assert that the caring is essentially, using Winnicott's (1945) concept, being a "good-enough" mother. They observe that in dementia care "a good-enough mother is not a perfect mother—just an ordinary person doing ordinary things" (p. 147). Further, they explain, "we believe that this, too, should be the whole procedure of dementia care: a steady presentation of the world to the person who has dementia; small manageable doses—small enough not to muddle, large enough to satisfy and be enjoyed; protection from complication; holding, handling, sharing. This is the fundamental role of the good-enough mother, or perhaps we should say good-enough dementia therapist, who is not perfect, not special, just an ordinary person, doing what, on the whole, comes naturally and intuitively" (p. 148).

Following are additional examples from the therapists interviewed on connecting and creating a holding environment.

"The longevity of the relationship is an important factor," says Scott Trudeau. "I work with the family dynamic and plant the seed for a long-term relationship with long-term goals and a long-term view. I have gotten involved and am moved. Then I know I have done my job. For example, when I go to a funeral, I send a card. That is an outcome measure of quality connection."

BEING TRUE TO SELF

Being able to be yourself is critical to being effective as a therapist. "You have to be real through occupation," says Scott Trudeau. "That is key, and students have to figure it out. It involves determining how to be comfortable and to focus on where the person is. On a very primitive level, the patient can sense the realness of the interaction. The interaction, the day-to-day work, is in carrying out the relationship. It is your responsibility to figure out how not to provoke. Good or bad, the occupational therapist is responsible.

"I will talk with the person who is afraid. I do reality testing with them," continues Trudeau. "I reality-test with everyone. I ask them, 'Will you be able to do it? Let us try it.' I try to build in success experiences. I mix some TLC with it and try to tap into the human aspect. I find out about their interests, such as a pet. I do a lot of psychiatric work."

MAKING THE CONNECTION

A great deal of what a therapist does with a client is developed through trial and error. "I think connecting with a patient very much takes place at the gut level and is based on experience," says Dalit Waller, OTR/L, with Neville Manor Nursing Home, an affiliate of Cambridge Somerville Health Alliance. "As a clinician, I have used many different approaches with people. I have tried a style and have had it backfire when I am really not connecting. So, I try other styles until we connect; it might not happen until mid-session, or I might not realize it until the end of a day, when I go back in my mind and think about the therapeutic relationship or about what tasks I might do differently in the future.

"Some people want you to be the expert, but most importantly [*sic*], they want you to be personal. It may involve getting them angry with you. They are, in fact, 'working' for you. I have seen inexperienced therapists try to get too technical, and they are not connecting with the patient. Many times, I do not even know what I have to do with the person in the first few sessions. It is not because I do not know what I am doing; I need to figure out what matters to the person; what is going on with the person."

BACK TO BASICS

One of the basic tools that therapists use is activity analysis. "I do it without thinking about it," says Waller. "I am looking at the different components. I am breaking everything down and adapting it. There is no one theory I adhere to. I think many theories make sense. The main thing is that what I do gets results. Gary Kielhofner's work [on the Model of Human Occupation], for example, makes a lot of sense to me; it is logical. No one likes to be seen in only one way. We are much more complicated than that. If people are more human in our eyes, we do a much better job with them. If we see someone as a competent homemaker rather than a frail woman in a johnny, we can connect to that person."

Some therapists describe interactive reasoning as having a continuum. "Residents, the clients, are getting good descriptions of what is to be expected in occupational therapy," says Sherlyn (Sherry) Fenton, OTR/L, of St. Camillus Health Center and Hospice, Whittingsville Massachusetts. "There should be a clear description of the role of OT, the clients' expected participation, and what will be the expected or desired outcomes. For example, outcomes might entail goal setting. It is actually an open dialogue between the patient and therapist. They discuss what is going on, what their priorities are, and so forth, so that appropriate goals can be set," says Fenton. "The person needs a clear idea of what the profession is about. It is all a part of getting the client to buy into the idea of occupational therapy. Once you can establish and maintain flow, clients can own their own program. They know it well enough and they are proud to tell others."

BEING PRESENT

Some therapists use interactive reasoning because it is an immediate feedback process. They also like its aspect of regard for the client, a practice that has its roots in the work of Carl Rogers. "It is critical to understand what the targets might be in terms of effecting affect," says Wally VanDyck. "It is also important to convey concern for clients' well-being as we work through the challenges. It is a constant process. You cannot be on automatic pilot—you cannot be thinking about what you are going to serve for dinner! You are constantly modifying and being attentive to the person. I think the consciousness of the process evolves with time and experience. The way I think of this is that the older generation is passing on things to the younger people. Experience is mentoring in the clinic. It is similar to how people whose native language is English do not think consciously about speaking English. You have learned the [grammar] rules, and you simply speak it. With clinical practice, after having studied learning theory and receiving structured supervision, co-teaching it is passing on culture."

EXPLORING AND INTERPRETING MOTIVES AS WELL AS OCCUPATION-BASED MEANINGS

Distancing in the therapeutic relationship is of particular concern as therapists work with an increasingly older client population and the necessity to ration health care services because of cost-containment measures. In addressing these concerns, Kautzmann (1993) demonstrates the importance of paying attention to the illness experience of the older adult and family through narrative reasoning. She proposes that through clients' stories, therapists create meaningful therapeutic interventions. It is as important for clients and families to tell stories as it is for therapists to listen to them, Kautzmann cautions. Therapists need to go beyond procedural reasoning to engage the older adult in treatment activities and for the activities to be therapeutic. She also warns that "power and control issues" are particularly salient in home health care, where the client has more power and control than he or she would have in an acute care setting.

Loss of roles, possessions and home, and relationships are significant issues for the elderly population. Health professionals also have less time to spend with clients. The emotional significance of role loss is particularly poignant in the chapter opening case study. The wife, now the caregiver, relied on her husband for over fifty years to shovel the driveway. Now her husband is unable to care for her. To protect his safety, she has to accept his limitations and give up both hope of change and a formerly need-satisfying, mutually dependent relationship.

In the following narratives, the therapists talk about getting to know the client. Their aim is to help the person move forward in a way that is meaningful to the person.

"I think first of all the therapist's task is getting to know the patient, how well he or she was doing," says Wally VanDyck. "During that process, it is essential to establish a comfort level and a rapport. We work toward clients' seeing me as an ally in getting them out of the hospital and moving things forward. It is necessary to understand the person's needs rather than have a preconceived agenda. The therapist is looking to prepare the person for the next step."

While connecting with a client starts with getting to know the person, it goes beyond the superficial when the therapist takes control of the relationship. "Establishing rapport with the older client on a personal level is my first goal," says Laura (Guertin) Impemba, OTR/L, of Health South Braintree and Pediatric Rehabilitation, Melrose, Massachuetts. "I try to adapt myself and reflect back the person's mood, but at the same time I am trying to alter it in order to engage the person. Depending upon the dynamics, I might be trying to gently encourage the person. I try to get the person engaged in a non–therapy-based conversation at first. I think it is particularly important to get out of the non-medical environment. I try to break up the routine and take the critical first five minutes to get to know the person. Then you have hopefully [*sic*] established rapport a little."

Listening

Listening involves sensing the other person. The following examples illustrate how listening is a strong value for the therapist.

"I think [therapeutic listening] is totally intuitive," says Turner. "For whatever reason, therapists have acquired excellent observation skills. Quietness about them allows them to understand and relate to the person in front of them. They are the ultimate caregiver; they can sense the other person. It might be a smile at the right time or a matter of pacing, tone, acceptance, and tolerance."

To enter the world of the person with dementia, caregivers must, while understanding the person's new world, give up their own sense of "order and form" (Perrin & May, 2000, p. 80). Perrin and May further explain that as the dementia progresses, there is an increased need for "reunion" between mother (figure) and the impaired person (pp. 56–57). This also requires that the activities match the well-being of the person and what is right for him or her in the here and now. Whether intuitive or not, the occupational therapist must act in a manner that is supportive and enables well-being at the client's level of ability. Using interactive reasoning can help a therapist gain control of his or her actions and words.

In working with older adults and caregivers, special attention needs to be given to conveying acceptance through listening. Perrin and May's observations directly capture the process of active listening at its best. There is the sensing of the other person and expression of acceptance that is both meaningful and understood by the caregiver and care receiver.

Understanding and Use of Narrative/Symbolic

The role of narrative and the symbolic with the older population is similar to reports of their use in the hospital setting. As stated earlier, stories told by the client and family are invaluable. Objects are essential cues to understanding the person and a focus of interactive reasoning. These understandings, therapists maintain, are necessary to establishing a collaborative relationship.

In the following example, the therapist speaks about the importance of objects and environment as symbols of the person. Institutions are home to many older adults. The few personal objects that remain are a valued source of information for the therapist's interactive reasoning.

Using Observational Skills

"Looking for clues in the objects in his or her room gives you an immediate sense of the person's support system," says Laura Impemba. "All of these things are key to telling you what is going on in this person's life."

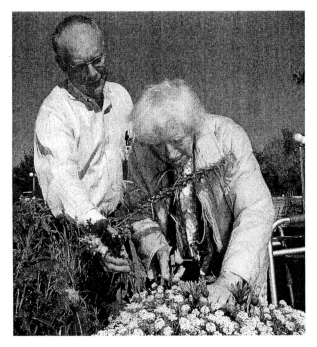

FIGURE 9.2 Use of the Symbolic in Creating a Relationship

BACK TO THE SUPPORT GROUP FOR CAREGIVERS

The therapist's reflections are the therapist's story. Although the therapist reassures himself that he is experienced, his narrative exposes a wish to establish credibility with the group. The therapist reminds himself that he is twenty years younger than the youngest group member, that the twelve caregivers are female, and that all of them have direct experience providing daily care for a loved one with dementia. The therapist wisely uses these self-reflections to strategize and reason about how he will interact with the group. He employs techniques such as humor and conveys to the members that they are the experts. The therapist is successful in establishing a forum for members to be of support to each other by learning from his narrative and self-analysis.

The experience of loss of significant occupations and objects is sometimes symbolized in a metaphor. In the chapter opening case study, and in the therapist's reflections, the loss of roles and the resultant grieving process are illustrated. The snowblower becomes the metaphor for loss and change in the client, family, support group, and therapist narratives. The following is a report of the therapist's experience.

"The client was help-rejecting in her style," says Scott Trudeau. "What happened in the end were multiple follow-ups. Ultimately, I got the son involved. He removed the snowblower and got the house plowed. On the unit, probably the majority of interaction is with the patients. However, it is easier to talk about the family because with the patient the interaction is so much more primitive. It is more difficult to talk about something that may appear very nonsensical that is meaningful to the patient and me. It is the relationship where the money is in being therapeutic with the patient.

"I facilitated the group to rescue me," continues Trudeau. "Before I shared my perspective, I had the group share their stories. The group goal is to validate. So as not to alienate the individual initially, the therapist brings in the group. This gave me time to organize and share some thoughts. That way, I had some validation before I confronted an individual. Safety is the group leader's responsibility, establishing trust, an atmosphere for disclosure, and concrete assurances of physical safety. Safety is the main job. It is physical safety in terms of snow plowing, even the emotional safety in the group context. (See Critical Case Questions 9.4 and 9.5.) The main issue was the dependency of the wife, according to the children. For her it was death, her husband's inability not to allow her to use the snowblower. Basically, we walked around her and let others [the family] do the snow plowing. Social work titrates the cyclical grieving. This is a major grief for the patient. For him to give up the 'macho thing' means she is confronting a major loss. The denial is 'he is not deteriorating, he is still in control.'" (See Critical Case Questions 9.6 and 9.7.)

SUMMARY

More attention needs to be paid to wellness as we consider models of interactive reasoning with the elderly population. Perrin and May's (2000) description of caring strategies for the older adult with dementia is fully consistent with the interactive reasoning themes and techniques described throughout this book. This gives good reason to consider caring occupational therapy practice with the older adult as a model for all practice. In light of the growing proportion of older adults, interactive reasoning with this group needs greater attention in education and practice. The roles of team members, as within any practice setting, influence the occupational therapist's education and ultimate modes of interactive reasoning.

New models such as peer support groups and wellness groups require the occupational therapist to study avenues for interactive reasoning from a group perspective. The large age span within the older years and social problems currently affecting the elderly are also looming issues. Community programs such as those for the homeless elderly require sophisticated clinical reasoning, as the functional problems are multidimensional. Finally, the complexities of interactive reasoning with the older population need to be considered from the perspective of the variety of settings, from home to community, hospital, rehabilitation program, and long-term care facility.

REFLECTIVE QUESTIONS

- What are your expectations of yourself as a daughter or son, niece or nephew, or grandchild in relation to the older adults in your family, and how might these expectations influence your work with this population?
- What are your expectations of yourself as a caregiver, and how might they influence your work with older adults and other caregivers?
- What other roles, if any, do you assume in caregiving with older adults in your community? What are the relationships like? Is this experience different from your actual or projected role as therapist?

- Imagine yourself as an older adult past sixty-five years of age. What would your life be like? How would you like to spend your time or wish to occupy yourself? What relationships would you have or desire? How might these perceptions influence your work with elderly individuals, their family, or caretakers?

INFORMATION CHECKPOINTS

9.1. INTERVENTION FORMATS IN WORKING WITH THE ELDERLY POPULATION

- One-to-one
- Couples
- Family
- Group
- Consultation

9.2. THERAPISTS' SPECIAL SKILLS

With a family or couple

- Understanding family and couples as systems with a dynamic balance.
- Acting with the knowledge that intervention can foster equilibrium or further disequilibrium in a couple or family system.

With a group

- Understanding small and large groups as systems with dynamics and processes.
- Acting with the knowledge that the leader role and processes vary in accordance with the centrality of purpose, be it educational, supportive, or change oriented.

9.3. THERAPIST ROLES

- Educator
- Consultant
- Therapist

9.4. ACTIVITY GOALS IN CAREGIVING AS PERCEIVED BY THE LAY FAMILY CAREGIVER (HASSELKUS, 1989, P. 649)

- Getting things done
- Achieving a sense of health and well-being for the care receiver
- Achieving a sense of health and well-being for the caregiver

CRITICAL CASE QUESTIONS

9.1. The occupational therapist describes his support group for caregivers. What are the potential benefits for the participants?

9.2. What roles does the group leader play in the group?

9.3. What leadership skills does he employ?

9.4. What is the therapist's story of the group? How did the plot change over the session described?

9.5. What is the group's story as a support group? How might the plot have changed in the group's story of itself?

9.6. What is the wife's story about her husband and the snowblower? How did the plot change during the session described?

9.7. What are the son's and the other children's stories about their father and the snowblower? How did the plot change for them after the therapist intervened?

KEY TERMS

DISTANCING

Not listening or attending to another person's feelings, anxieties, and pain demonstrated in one's behavior, attitudes, or inaction. This may be conscious or unconsciously driven.

GROUP DYNAMICS AND PROCESS

The forces and actions that influence a group at the level of the individual, the subgroup, and the group as a whole.

SMALL GROUPS

Groups usually composed of no more than eight or ten members.

LARGE GROUPS

Groups usually composed of ten or more members. They can range from midsize, ten to twenty-five people, to extremely large, more than twenty-five people.

EDUCATION AND RESEARCH

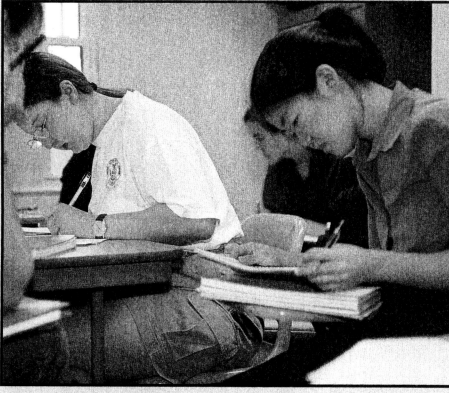

PART IV

Interactive Reasoning Requires Qualitative Analysis of Narrative

*T*he book concludes in chapter 10 with attention given to education and research. The field's maturation is dependent upon both the next generation of therapists and verification of the occupational therapy practice. There is great skepticism among therapists that therapeutic relationship skills, considered by many to be intuitive, can be taught. The author defeats this position.

By drawing upon her experience as an educator and the works of her colleagues, the author outlines teaching strategies for developing clinical reasoning skills in occupational therapy students and practitioners. She gives special attention to guiding the development of interactive reasoning skills. It is fitting to devote the last pages of the text to research. Much has been written since clinical reasoning was first described in occupational therapy. In summarizing over fifteen years of work, the author ends with questions for future inquiry.

APPLICATIONS TO EDUCATION AND CURRENT RESEARCH

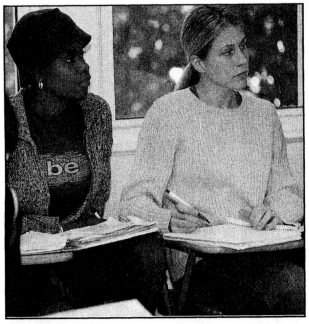

FIGURE 10.1   Developing the Language of Interactive Reasoning Thought Processes at Tufts University, Boston School of Occupational Therapy

STUDENT IN THE CLINIC
By Pina Masciarelli-Patel
(March 6, 2000)

CASE STUDY 10.1

On the first day of a level I affiliation, a student approached me somewhat anxious and annoyed that a client had repeatedly asked him personal questions. The questions were "Where do you live?" and "Do you like Fleetwood Mac?" The student wondered, "Why does she keep asking me the same questions over and over? She won't stop!" I suggested to the student that he reflect on his own question. At first, the student thought the client just needed to know his personal business. However, with encouragement to use a phenomenological approach, the student was able to move toward the client's own worries of having "another new person" in the program. With this understanding, the student explored the client's concerns from the client's

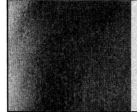

perspective. The student then returned to the classroom. The client with the same questions soon approached him. Armed with his new insights, the student initiated a discussion about what it was like to have a new person in the program. The client took part in this brief interaction and not only walked away with ease but also did not ask any other questions. The student returned very excited about his first intervention.

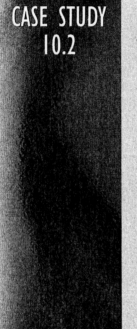

CASE STUDY 10.2

STUDENT IN THE UNIVERSITY
By Pina Masciarelli-Patel
(March 6, 2000)

A first-year master's student completed a videotaped peer interview for an initial class assignment. The student was quite pleased with herself. She had followed her script exactly and discovered many similarities between herself and the interviewee: similar cultural backgrounds, leisure interests, educational backgrounds, plans for marriage and families, and common career focuses. The student felt that she had obtained the interviewee's perspective and had conducted a thorough interview. However, what the student had failed to do was to ask the interviewee what was meaningful to her, what were her goals, her accomplishments, etc. The questions were closed and direct, with the student focusing on what she and the interviewee had in common. The student did recognize that the interviewee had a "blank expression," "sat motionless," and answered many questions with one-word answers. However, she was unable to connect this to the interview process. Although the student was quite pleased with her results, what she missed was the purpose of the occupational therapy interview—establishing what was meaningful to her client.

OVERVIEW

*T*he previous chapters presented the philosophy, borrowed theory and practice, and interactive reasoning of occupational therapists in practice. This chapter addresses both academic and clinical education of the occupational therapist. It summarizes the progress made in studying problems related to interactive reasoning in occupational therapy.

This chapter gives particular emphasis to the development of interactive reasoning and therapeutic relating skills. A need exists to pay attention to the differences between the novice and expert practitioner (McKay & Ryan, 1995; Robertson, 1996) in the models of education provided. A review of the state of research in the realm of interactive reasoning demonstrates growing interest and a need for further study. As one can see in the chapter opening case studies, both students, as novices, erred by an absence of attention to the other person's frame of reference. Further, because the scope of the other person was narrow, the students were not making use of evidence-based research data and patterns in their own experience.

EDUCATION OF THE OCCUPATIONAL THERAPIST

CLINICAL REASONING AS A MODEL FOR EDUCATION

Tufts University initiated a curriculum design in 1986 that focused on developing clinical reasoning abilities in its entry-level master student graduates. It was the first of its kind. The curriculum was structured around Fleming and Mattingly's recent research discovery of forms of reasoning in occupational therapy that included procedural, interactive, conditional, and narrative dimensions (Cohen, 1993). Neistadt's creation of "classroom as a clinic model" was introduced and incorporated into the program. This model has been detailed in the occupational therapy literature (Neistadt, 1987, 1992).

There were four core courses in the Tufts model: observation, interactive reasoning, procedural reasoning, and analytical reasoning. The interactive reasoning course, of particular relevance here, built on students' observation skills. The students learned how to develop a narrative based upon interviews with guest speakers telling of their illness or disability experience. The curriculum continues to this day to build upon the original model set forth over fifteen years ago. It has been met with great success. There have been both informal and formal (Neistadt, 1992, 1998) reports of the effectiveness of using clinical reasoning as a thinking frame in occupational therapy curriculum.

DEVELOPING NARRATIVE REASONING ABILITY

The narrative approach has much to offer in the basic and advanced education of an occupational therapist. It involves meaning making that according to Chapparo and Ranka (2000) has two dimensions: "meaning schemes" and "meaning perspectives." Ryan (1999) points out that stories can help students build their own personal theories about practice and, with help, use them to see the larger picture as well as the details. (See Information Checkpoint 10.1.)

PERSONAL KNOWLEDGE AND STRESS MANAGEMENT

Personal knowledge is particularly relevant to clinical reasoning in health professions (Higgs & Titchen, 2000, pp. 28–29). Higgs and Titchen believe that this type of knowledge is unique to an individual's sense of self and internal frame of reference and results from personal experience and reflection. They explain, "The individual's behaviour is highly influenced by his/her frame of reference. Within this frame of reference, scientific knowledge and professional knowledge are translated into decisions for practice which are influenced by the individual's convictions and judgements about the worth of this knowledge and its relevance to the current situation. New knowledge is compared with the individual's existing system of beliefs and values. If new knowledge or ideas are incongruent with their belief system, individuals may reject the new information" (pp. 28–29).

Personal knowledge can help the student as well as the practitioner modulate the stress inherent in the work of helping and can help prevent burnout. Interpersonal situations are bound to raise issues for the therapist, and the helping role is bound to be emotionally depleting. It is critical that students explore and reflect upon their own belief systems early in the education process. (See Critical Case Questions 10.1 and 10.2.) The therapist's internal frame of reference will ultimately be the screen to interpret and direct the course of interventions (Chapparo & Ranka, 2000). External stresses such as role ambiguity and role conflict also can lead to professional burnout (Davis, 1998). Students will benefit from learning ways to intervene and prevent burnout, such as use of time management skills, vacations, peer as well as supervisory support, and good communication.

There have been reports that occupational therapists do not use narrative reasoning as much as they use procedural reasoning. It has been recommended that educational programs look for ways to foster this capability and the use of various forms of clinical reasoning (Alnervik & Sviden, 1996; Gitlin, Corcoran, & Leinmiller-Eckhardt, 1995; Hallin & Sviden, 1995; McKay & Ryan, 1995; Neistadt & Atkins, 1996; Schwartz, 1991). (See Critical Case Question 10.3.)

One strategy for further promoting the development of clinical reasoning skills calls for making the language of clinical reasoning thought processes more explicit in teaching (Neistadt, 1996) and for the use of "interactive journals" (Tryssenaar, 1995) to promote reflection. The use of collaborative models such as interdisciplinary education (MacKinnon, 1996), teaching tools like written clinical reasoning case studies (Neistadt, Wight, & Mulligan, 1998), videotapes (Cohen, 1989; Crepeau, 1991), and computer interactive simulations (Tomlin & Stone, 1997) has also been suggested as a means to enhancing clinical reasoning abilities. (See Critical Case Question 10.4.) Strategies for teaching technical skills along with reasoning in fieldwork education (Cohen, 1989) as well as staff development and retention through analysis of practice have also been proposed (Slater & Cohen, 1991). Problem-based learning is commonly reported as a model for promoting clinical reasoning skills in occupational therapy and other fields of practice.

PROBLEM-BASED LEARNING

Various formats of problem-based learning have been proposed as a means to teach clinical reasoning. Royeen (1995) offered a problem-based learning curriculum that aimed to foster competencies for health care in the twenty-first century. She purported that the problem-based curriculum would prepare practitioners in clinical reasoning and critical reflection as well as in clinical skills and technical knowledge. VanLeit (1995) suggested the use of case method to enhance problem solving and reasoning ability in an occupational therapy curriculum.

Dudgeon and Greenberg (1998) support the use of problem-based learning as a way to expose students to the complex and diverse issues in consultation roles. They view issues related to knowledge, interpersonal skills, and diversity readiness as essential to the new practitioner's ability to act as a consultant. The knowledge includes standards of practice, frames of reference, evidence-based practice, and practice settings and systems (p. 803). The interpersonal skills include communication, partnership, leadership, negotiation, education, and training (p. 803). Diversity readiness includes community, cultural, and resource systems (p. 803).

MULTICULTURAL SENSITIVITY

It has been suggested that the occupational therapist's view of reality influences how the practitioner frames clinical practice (Hooper, 1997). According to Hooper, this view includes beliefs about ultimate reality, life, death, and eternity, human nature, and the nature of knowing. Yuen and Matthew (1999) point out that multicultural awareness and sensitivity have been advocated in the occupational therapy literature. They found that experiential learning by interviewing a person of a different ethnic background can improve awareness and to some extent sensitivity and attitude toward another cultural group.

Crepeau (1991) points out that educators need to encourage students to see the importance of beliefs and values held by clients so that a better balance is achieved between professional power and the client's experience. In Case Study 10.1, the occupational therapy student and his client were both distraught. Each lacked an understanding of the other's values and concerns. Interestingly, rather than seeing the commonality, both felt uncomfortable with newness in a situation, but from the perspective of their separate roles. Once the issues were explored, the parallel features in their stories brought the opportunity for empathic connection.

VALUE OF EXPERIENTIAL LEARNING

Although educators value theory, for many it is the integration of actual experience with theory and self-reflection that produces a strong practitioner. Molly Campbell, OTR/L, of the Brookline Public Schools, Perkins School for the Blind, and part-time instructor at Tufts University, Boston School of Occupational Therapy, gives her perspective through her observations from her own career as a therapist and instructor. Campbell notes, "At this point, interactive reasoning feels like intuition. I would say theories, but I almost forget the theories. I am vague about the schools of thought. I don't use the word, but I translate it, like Kielhofner. It feels like intuition, like a commonsense after all these years, but it is backed up by a theory or a therapeutic rationale. I could tease out all the science when I have to. I really do not think about Kielhofner, but his name is out there. I learned most from experience and so little from school. I would have more level-one observations. I would build up the requirements for experience of the relationship. I would include as many opportunities to interact one on one implementing activities with clients and being a PCA [personal care attendant]. It doesn't matter what it is about as long as they [students or applicants] are really interacting with the person, where they are investing a little bit of themselves into the interaction, where they are responsible."

Deborah Rochman, OTR/L, also a part-time instructor at Tufts University, Boston School of Occupational Therapy, and in private practice as an occupational therapist, emphasizes the value of actual experience in learning. She says, "It is a process you have to live through because so much of it is psychodynamic in supervision. Experience as a practitioner is something you have to go through and process with someone else. Seeing other people interview is also valuable."

Herself an experienced clinician and assistant professor at Tufts University, Boston School of Occupational Therapy, Sharon Ray, OTR/L, also emphasizes the necessity for a lot of clinical experience in education. She remarks, "Education of the therapist—a lot is clinical experience. I always felt reading someone's cues was helpful. Part of that comes with practice and experience. Try to check back with the person and see if the intervention is validated. I read cues, practice, and validate for myself if the cues are correct. I always had clear guidelines and expectations [in family, father was in the military]. That clearness comes from that background. That desire for clarity comes from my teaching."

RESEARCH

For the past fifteen years, the research and writing on clinical reasoning in occupational therapy have flourished since early reports such as the one by Gillete and Mattingly (1987). In concluding this book, it is relevant to look at what we now know about interactive reasoning in occupational therapy and related fields. It is also pertinent to examine areas needed for further research. As Tickle-Degnen (2000) concludes, there is a clear need for evidence-based research to enhance clinical reasoning in occupational therapy.

MODELS OF RESEARCH

Many models are used to study clinical reasoning in the health professions. (See Information Checkpoint 10.2.) Information-processing models and clinical reasoning studies in nursing and medicine serve as benchmarks for investigations in occupational therapy (Roberts, 1996). The explanations are based on investigations that are either process oriented or content (knowledge) oriented (Higgs & Jones, 2000). Higgs and Jones identify several interpretive models of clinical reasoning. (See Information Checkpoint 10.3 and Table 10.1.) Based upon interpretive paradigm research studies, the interpretive and critical paradigms are distinctly relevant to occupational therapy and are gaining prominence in the health fields (Higgs & Jones, 2000, p. 5). According to Higgs and Jones, Crepeau's and Fleming's work on structuring meaning and interpreting the problem from the client's perspective is an example of such research in occupational therapy.

TABLE 10.1	
INTERPRETIVE CLINICAL REASONING MODEL AND INFORMATION SOURCE*	
INTERPRETIVE MODEL	**INFORMATION SOURCE FOR THE THERAPIST**
Diagnostic reasoning	What are the impairment, disability, or handicap and the underlying pathobiological mechanism?
Interactive reasoning	How can the intervention be more effectively managed through interaction or social exchange?
Narrative reasoning	What stories about past or present patients can be told to further the current patient's understanding or manage an intervention?
Collaborative reasoning	What information should be actively sought from the client and used in shared decision making?
Conditional reasoning	Based on information ascertained, what is the therapist's estimation of the patient's response to intervention?
Ethical/pragmatic reasoning	What decisions are being made in the realm of ethical dilemmas related to moral, political, and economic concerns?
Teaching as reasoning	What information, guidance, or advice is the therapist consciously giving to promote change in the patient's behavior, understanding, or feelings?

*Summarized in tabular form from Higgs & Jones, 2000, p. 8.

Generally three types of research models are used in studying the interpretive perspective on interactive reasoning:

1. An ethnographic approach of learning from the whole narrative itself.
2. A qualitative analytic approach of categorizing concepts in advance of analysis.
3. A combined approach of coding concepts after discovering categories from narrative analysis and interpretation.

The purpose of this review is to act as a compass for giving direction to current practice and future research. As we discover and define practice, the outcomes of intervention can be better targeted and studied.

Rightfully there is overlap between fields using interpretive approaches, and studies from other disciplines offer insights from which we can learn. Nevertheless, as with any research, interpretive studies need examination. Patel and Arocha (2000) caution that these types of studies need to be examined because of two main unresolved issues. First, there is the need to clarify the purpose of such research. Second, there are questions about the generalizability of the findings. The latter concerns the potential artificiality of conditions severely distorting what would happen in real-life situations.

NARRATIVE PROCESS

Mattingly (1991b) believes that narrative reasoning is the central form of clinical reasoning in occupational therapy. She explains that this mode of reasoning is used when the therapist is concerned with how the disability or illness affects a person's life, what she calls the "illness experience."

Narrative reasoning has been used to explain variables related to successful practice. An analysis of therapist reflections on their practice revealed success factors related to school-based occupational therapy (Case-Smith, 1997). Telling the story of practice has also illuminated other aspects of practice. For example, it has revealed the complexities of pediatric-based practice and working with children's families (Medhurst & Ryan, 1996a, 1996b) and the meaning of caregiving for frail elderly people living in the community (Hasselkus, 1989), and it has aided our understanding of the illness experience of older adults and their families (Kautzmann, 1993). In addition to its value to understanding occupational therapy, narrative reasoning is considered of direct value to the client. In one study, narrative reasoning was speculated to have the potential to influence the illness experience of a person with cancer in terms of her beliefs, sense of control, and perceptions of the illness (Mostert, Zacharkiewicz, & Fossey, 1996).

McLeod and Balamoutsou (1996) were interested in studying a whole narrative to understand types of events in client-centered therapy. Recognizing its limitations, they chose to study a single session of therapy through a qualitative analysis of the narrative. The researchers identified five main types of narrative process:

1. *Embeddedness.* There is a core story that the client tells in the beginning. From this opening comes a series of stories that are embedded with meanings. Some of the stories are initiated by the client and others by the therapist. The story acts as a means for the client to move from one feeling state to another.
2. *Co-construction.* The therapist is active in construction of the narrative. Several methods are used as the therapist co-constructs the story. These

interventions include empathic reflection, therapist-as-chorus, therapist narrative elaboration, and therapist-provided metanarrative.

3. *Narrative tensions.* The creation of the narrative is around one main tension: the client's sense of how he was and his goal of how he would like to be. During the session the therapist and client search and test a variety of intentions and feeling states. The ultimate aim is to find a way to resolve the tension and complete the story.

4. *Point of view.* The client's point of view is told in a variety of ways that reflect the client's subjective world. Metaphors can be interpreted as a reflection of the client's subjective point of view.

5. *Narrative markers.* "Narrative markers are momentary verbal or nonverbal events or signals that serve to orient the listener to important features of the narrative flow. . . . These orientation markers appeared to locate stories within an overall life-history, and also to indicate an awareness of the needs of the listener and the information he would require to make sense of a story" (p. 71).

Through narrative analysis of a single therapy session, McLeod and Balamoutsou (1996) found the role and function of narrative. The session was made up of a series of embedded stories. Sometimes a recurring metaphor or image linked the meaning across stories. The authors found that using Riessman's (1993) two questions "What stories are being told here?" and "How are these stories being constructed?" revealed a deeper level of appreciation and understanding.

Rosa and Hasselkus (1996) studied the narratives of eighty-three therapists from a nationwide sample. The narratives were derived from "phenomenologic" telephone interviews conducted in a larger study. For the study, therapists were asked to describe experiences that were especially satisfying and dissatisfying in their practices. The purpose of this particular analysis was to understand the relationship between occupational therapists and their clients. Through a coded analysis of the transcripts, the researchers identified a broad category and related data clustered around subthemes. The broad core theme was "connecting with patients" (p. 248). The two subthemes were "helping patients" and "working together with patients" (p. 248). Throughout the analysis, the researchers used the constant comparative method to compare like coded text segments with each other and with information in the literature. They also used other strategies to ensure validity to their interpretations. These techniques included avoiding the use of a priori categories, sharing findings with colleagues, and frequent discussion between the researchers that focused on the lived experience rather than examination of the therapeutic process.

Further support is given in the literature to the importance of developing the art of reflecting on practice. Alnervik and Sviden (1996) studied occupational therapists' patterns of reflection on practice. They asked therapists to share narratives about their practice, that is, to "tell the story." They also asked them to share reflections on practice, that is, to describe the thinking around how they had conducted the treatment. They found that procedural reasoning was predominant in storytelling and reflection on practice. Further, they observed that few comments were classified as involving interactive or conditional reasoning. Alnervik and Sviden concluded that therapists need to develop their ability to use storytelling and be more attentive to the role of reflection in examining, teaching, and developing the art of occupational therapy.

As demonstrated in Case Study 10.2, problems in establishing rapport evolve when there is an absence of reflection. The student missed the interviewee's perspective because she followed a script. Rather than struggle with discerning meanings, she made initial assumptions solely based upon manifest content. The student's underlying motivation was her own need to please her professor by doing the "assignment" correctly. Such a misalliance brings with it the message to the client that the protocol is more important than the relationship and that being perfect is a possibility.

Alnervik and Sviden (1996) also found it of value to study comments as a unit of analysis versus submerging all the comments into the broad categories. The latter broad categories of analysis included procedural, interactive, and conditional reasoning. In an earlier study, Hallin and Sviden (1995) studied occupational therapists' reflections on practice in three different treatment sessions. These situations included self-care, preparing and eating food, and a home visit. Five types of comments were characteristic of the therapists' reflections: "confident, tentative, generalized, teaching, and understanding." The researchers concluded that in developing occupational therapy, different forms of reasoning should be explored.

CONTEXT OF PRACTICE

The former studies imply the influence of context or setting on therapist reasoning and reflections on practice. Based on their comprehensive review of the occupational therapy literature, Schell and Cervero (1993) strongly advised that contextual issues be considered in studying clinical reasoning. Contextual influences were also concluded to effect therapists' adopting a pragmatic or relativistic form of reasoning in community-based occupational therapy (Munroe, 1996).

In a study examining the differences between occupational therapists working in rheumatology and neurology, Sviden and Hallin (1999) did find differences in their clinical reasoning. The field of practice, the researchers speculate, may have influenced the therapist-patient relationship. It may also be the setting that defined the process. Program type and treatment site, in fact, have been found to account for differences in type of activity used—passive, enabling, versus purposeful activity—in occupational therapy interventions (Schell & Cervero, 1995). In the former study, the treatments were for adults with physical or cognitive impairments. The settings included acute inpatient, rehabilitation inpatient, and outpatient services at bedside, in the clinic, and in natural contexts. One should also consider the influence of therapist values on the clinical reasoning process in occupational therapy (Fondiller, Rosage, & Neuhaus, 1990).

In a pilot study, Toth-Cohen (2000) examined occupational therapists' role perceptions as providers of education and support for caregivers of individuals with dementia. Using descriptive interviews, she found several themes that reflect the importance influence of the family perspective in the home environment. In regard to interaction, her study strongly suggests that occupational therapists working with caregivers listen, accept the lay caregiver as expert, validate the efforts of the caregiver, assist the caregiver to transfer known strategies to other problematic areas, and reframe the situation of caregiving by seeing the situation in a different way. Reframing usually included giving permission to caretakers to take time for themselves, to give up expectations of themselves and the family member with dementia that were no longer working, and to assume a different standard to judge the merits of their strategies.

COLLABORATING WITH THE CLIENT

Rosa and Hasselkus (1996) studied therapist helping. Their findings bear close resemblance to what therapists told me in the interviews conducted for this book and what I found in the occupational therapy literature. They found that *"helping as connecting* was defined as therapists' perceptions that they had provided some aspect of patient care that was valued by patients and that resulted in outcomes meaningful to patients" (p. 249). Other aspects of helping included the therapists' "sense of personal ownership of what happened to their patients," "getting patients to see," that is, getting them to take note of and value their progress, and "being there" in the sense of offering support and comfort (p. 250). The concept of working together involved sharing the work and the responsibilities of the therapy, doing together, which included problem solving and formulating goals, and pooling resources in the sense of the therapist and patient offering mutual support and enthusiasm in sharing the work of the therapy (pp. 251–252). The researchers concluded that doing the work therapy required the occupational therapist to combine personal and professional identities. In sum, "the essence of the concept of working together with patients was a sense of joining together in mutually supportive partnerships characterized by compatibility, reciprocity, and rapport" (p. 251).

Client collaboration in the therapeutic process cuts across practice settings and populations. The process begins in the first contact. One study bears directly on this point. Mew and Fossey (1996) conducted a single case study using the Canadian Occupational Performance Measure to examine the client-centered aspects of clinical reasoning. Their findings suggest that during assessment, collaboration in process of defining problems and negotiating intervention goals was central to the client-centered clinical reasoning. The therapist used three main approaches: (1) collaboration to define problems and to negotiate therapy goals to arrive at mutually agreeable views—this involved providing "expert" information to help the client make informed choices, (2) acknowledgment of the client's feelings by the therapist, and (3) understanding of the client by the therapist. Several questions were left unanswered: Does the therapist provide information as to whether he or she agrees with the client's decision? Does the therapist make his or her own decisions when considering the client's view? To what extent does the therapist collaborate, and how consistent is it?

In both case studies opening this chapter, the students lacked an understanding of the other person's story. They focused on the procedural aspects of the interaction rather than explore meaning within an occupational context. Here were missed opportunities to form connections and collaborative relationships. The research reviewed clearly indicates that we broaden students' ability to use a variety of forms of clinical reasoning, interactive and narrative reasoning being underemployed by therapists.

The degree of attention to the themes and techniques generated by this author's research is growing (see Table 10.2). The emphasis in the research literature given to each of the areas is uneven and in some instances nonexistent. However, therapist reports do portray a coherent picture that suggests that the themes are meaningful. Further inquiry is recommended because of these narrative reports, anecdotal information, and the existing literature.

TABLE 10.2	
INTERACTIVE REASONING RESEARCH	
THEMES	**RELATIVE DEGREE OF ATTENTION***
Active participation and collaboration	H
Engaging/connecting and creating a holding environment	M
Exploring/interpreting motives and occupation-based meanings	M
Listening	L
Understanding and use of narrative/symbolic	H
TECHNIQUES	
Selling	H
Giving back	L
Engaging the mood	L
Validating	M
Holding	M

*H = high, M = medium, L = low to none

BACK TO THE STUDENTS IN THE CLINIC AND THE UNIVERSITY

In both case studies, the occupational therapy students benefited from direct experience and reflection. Through an analysis of interactions they were able to identify strategies to alter their interventions. Seeing the situation from the perspective of the person they were helping enabled the reasoning process to progress.

SUMMARY

Interactive reasoning has been demonstrated to be a productive and fruitful area of research. Outcome studies will add to our understanding of both the theory and practice of interactive reasoning. As a component of the broader notion of clinical reasoning, interactive reasoning serves as a solid model for educating future practitioners. Crabtree (1998) questions whether therapists do in fact use different forms of reasoning. She asks whether in the literature we are using a variety of images to explain and put into words a phenomenon that is tacit. Whether interactive reasoning can or should be teased out from other forms of clinical reasoning is left open to debate. Nevertheless, future investigations into interactive reasoning are indicated.

REFLECTIVE QUESTIONS

- Many interpretive models of clinical reasoning are described in the literature. Would you find them of equal value in working with different populations and settings? Explain your rationale.

- There are varying time frames for intervention. What, if any, influence do they have for the type(s) of reasoning employed? In reflecting upon your own pace, are you better suited for therapeutic relationships that are short-term or long-term, and why?
- What do you surmise are the reasons for therapists neglecting interactive and narrative reasoning approaches over other forms of reasoning such as procedural reasoning?
- Narratives are suggested as useful to developing the art of practice in occupational therapy. Imagine starting your own reflective journal on your experiences as a novice, intermediate, or expert practitioner. Identify an audience and tell the story. Who are the actors? What is the plot? What is untold? What story is, for example, the client, student, family member, or teacher in? What are the "narrative tensions" and "narrative markers"?

INFORMATION CHECKPOINTS

10.1. DISCOURSE

"Practitioners need fluency in the discourse about pain and courage, and that discourse requires the capacity to think and feel at once" (Peloquin, 1995, p. 25).

10.2. MODELS OF CLINICAL REASONING

Models that explain and interpret clinical reasoning process include hypothetico-deductive, pattern recognition, knowledge reasoning integration or interaction between knowledge and skills, reasoning as a process of integrating knowledge, cognition, and metacognition, and interpretive (Higgs & Jones, 2000).

10.3. INTERPRETIVE MODELS OF CLINICAL REASONING (HIGGS & JONES, 2000, P. 8)

- Diagnostic reasoning
- Interactive reasoning
- Narrative reasoning
- Collaborative reasoning
- Predictive or conditional reasoning
- Ethical/pragmatic reasoning
- Teaching as reasoning

CRITICAL CASE QUESTIONS

10.1. As fieldwork supervisor, you would like your student in the clinic (Case Study 10.1) to be able to perceive the client's point of view. What questions would you suggest the student ask himself to get a better understanding of the client's concerns? What is the student's story? What is the client's story?

10.2. The occupational therapy student in the clinic comes to understand that the personal questions reflect the client's anxiety about newcomers and her fear of closeness. What techniques would be appropriate to use to form a connection with the client? What is your reasoning?

10.3. The student in the university (Case Study 10.2) was frustrated with the comments on her assignment. She believed she had thoroughly gathered the background information. What forms of clinical reasoning would you suggest the student use? What type of information would they yield?

10.4. What strategies can the university student use to develop her own self-understanding and to establish what is meaningful to her interviewee?

KEY TERMS

HYPOTHETICO-DEDUCTIVE REASONING

Often linked to procedural reasoning in occupational therapy, it is the generation of hypotheses based upon clinical data and knowledge and the testing of these hypotheses through further inquiry—the "if . . . then" mode (Higgs & Jones, 2000, pp. 5–6).

MEANING PERSPECTIVES

"Meaning perspectives are made up of higher-order schemata, theories and beliefs. They refer to the structure of assumptions and beliefs within which a new experience is interpreted" (Chapparo & Ranka, 2000, p. 134).

MEANING SCHEMES

"Meaning schemes are sets of related and habitual expectations governing if/then relationships" (Chapparo & Ranka, 2000, p. 133).

METACOGNITION

"Being aware of one's cognitive processes and exerting control over these processes, and the cognitive skills that are necessary for the management of knowledge and other cognitive skills" (Higgs & Jones, 2000, p. 9).

REFERENCES

Alnervik, A., & Sviden, G. (1996). On clinical reasoning: Patterns of reflection on practice. *Occupational Therapy Journal of Research, 16*(2), 98–110.

American Occupational Therapy Association (AOTA). (1999). Standards of practice for occupational therapy, AOTA, 1998. *American Journal of Occupational Therapy, 53*(3), 294–295.

American Occupational Therapy Association (AOTA). (1999). The guide to occupational therapy practice. *American Journal of Occupational Therapy, 53*(3), 247–322.

Anderson, R., & Cissna, K. (1997). *The Martin Buber-Carl Rogers dialogue: A new transcript with commentary.* Albany: State University of New York Press.

Borg, B., & Bruce, M. A. (1991). *The group system: The therapeutic activity group in occupational therapy.* Thorofare, NJ: Slack.

Borg, B., & Bruce, M. A. (1997). *Occupational therapy stories: Psychosocial interaction in practice.* Thorofare, NJ: Slack.

Bradburn, S. L. (1992). *Psychiatric occupational therapists' strategies for engaging patients in treatment during the initial interview.* Unpublished master's thesis, Tufts University, Medford, MA.

Buber, M. (1965). *The knowledge of man: Selected essays* (M. Friedman & R. G. Smith, Trans.; M. Friedman, Ed.). New York: Harper and Row.

Buber, M. (1970). *I and thou* (Originally written in 1922) (W. Kaufmann, Trans.). New York: Macmillan.

Case-Smith, J. (1997). Variables related to successful school-based practice. *Occupational Therapy Journal of Research, 17*(2), 133–153.

Chapparo, C., & Ranka, J. (2000). Clinical reasoning in occupational therapy. In J. Higgs & M. Jones (Eds.), *Clinical reasoning in the health professions* (2nd ed.) (pp. 128–137). Oxford: Butterworth-Heinemann.

Christiansen, C. H. (1999). Defining lives: Occupation as identity: An essay on competence, coherence, and the creation of meaning. *American Journal of Occupational Therapy, 53*(6), 547–558.

Clark, F. (1993). Occupation embedded in a real life: Interweaving occupational science and occupational therapy. 1993 Eleanor Clarke Slagle lecture. *American Journal of Occupational Therapy, 47*(12), 1067–1078.

Cohn, E. S. (1989). Fieldwork education: Shaping a foundation for clinical reasoning. *American Journal of Occupational Therapy, 43*(4), 240–244.

Cohn, E. S. (1991). Clinical reasoning: Explicating complexity. *American Journal of Occupational Therapy, 45*, 969–971.

Cohn, E. S. (1993). Inquiring minds: A curriculum designed to facilitate clinical reasoning. *Education Special Interest Section Newsletter, American Occupational Therapy Association, 3*(4), 1–2.

Cole, M. B. (1998). *Group dynamics in occupational therapy: The theoretical basis and practice application of group treatment* (2nd ed.). Thorofare, NJ: Slack.

Combs, A. W., Avila, D. L., & Purkey, W. W. (1971). *Helping relationships: Basic concepts for the helping professions.* Boston: Allyn and Bacon.

Crabtree, M. (1998). Images of reasoning: A literature review. *Australian Occupational Therapy Journal, 45*(4), 113–123.

Creighton, C., Dijkers, M., Bennett, N., & Brown, K. (1995). Reasoning and the art of therapy for spinal cord injury. *American Journal of Occupational Therapy, 49*(4), 311–317.

Crepeau, E. B. (1991). Achieving intersubjective understanding: Examples from an occupational therapy treatment session. *American Journal of Occupational Therapy, 45*(11), 1016–1025.

Csikszentmihalyi, M. (1975). *Beyond boredom and anxiety. The experience of play in work and games.* San Francisco: Jossey-Bass.

Csikszentmihalyi, M. (1990). *Flow: The psychology of optimal experience.* New York: Harper and Row.

Csikszentmihalyi, M. (1993). *The evolving self: A psychology for the third millennium.* New York: HarperCollins.

Csikszentmihalyi, M. (1996). *Creativity flow and the psychology of discovery and invention.* New York: HarperCollins.

Csikszentmihalyi, M., & Csikszentmihalyi, I. S. (1988). *Optimal experience: Psychological studies of flow in consciousness.* Cambridge: Cambridge University Press.

Davidson, D., & Peloquin, S. M. (1998). *Making connections with others: A handbook on interpersonal practice.* Bethesda, MD: American Occupational Therapy Association.

Davis, C. M. (1998). *Patient practitioner interaction: An experiential manual for developing the art of health care* (3rd ed.). Thorofare, NJ: Slack.

Dudgeon, B. J., & Greenberg, S. L. (1998). Preparing students for consultation roles and systems. *American Journal of Occupational Therapy, 52*(1), 801–809.

Duncombe, L. W., Howe, M. C., & Schwartzberg, S. L. (1988). *Case simulations in psychosocial occupational therapy* (2nd ed.). Philadelphia: F. A. Davis.

Egan, G. (1982). *The skilled helper: Model, skills, and methods for effective helping* (2nd ed.). Monterey, CA: Brooks/Cole.

Erikson, E. H. (1984). Reflections on the last stage—and the first. *Psychoanalytic Study of the Child, 39,* 155–165.

Evenson, M., & Roberts, P. (1996). A clinical reasoning model for working with individuals who have had a stroke. In C. B. Royeen (Ed.), *STROKE: Strategies, treatment, rehabilitation, outcomes, knowledge, and evaluation,* Lesson 4 of AOTA's self-paced clinical course (pp. 1–50). Bethesda, MD: American Occupational Therapy Association.

Fazio, L. (1992). Tell me a story: The therapeutic metaphor in the practice of pediatric occupational therapy. *American Journal of Occupational Therapy, 46*(2), 112–119.

Fidler, G. S., & Fidler, J. W. (1963). *Occupational therapy: A communication process in psychiatry.* New York: Macmillan.

Fidler, G. S., & Fidler, J. W. (1978). Doing and becoming: Purposeful action and self-actualization. *American Journal of Occupational Therapy, 32*(5), 305–310.

Fleming, M. H. (1991a). Clinical reasoning in medicine compared with clinical reasoning in occupational therapy. *American Journal of Occupational Therapy, 45,* 988–996.

Fleming, M. H. (1991b). The therapist with the three-track mind. *American Journal of Occupational Therapy, 45,* 1007–1014.

Fleming, M. H. (1993). Aspects of clinical reasoning in occupational therapy. In H. Hopkins & H. Smith (Eds.), *Willard and Spackman's occupational therapy* (8th ed.) (pp. 867–880). Philadelphia: J. B. Lippincott.

Fleming, M. H. (1994). The therapist with the three-track mind. In C. Mattingly and M. H. Fleming, *Clinical reasoning: Forms of inquiry in therapeutic practice* (pp. 119–136). Philadelphia: F. A. Davis.

Fleming, M. H., & Mattingly, C. (1994). Giving language to practice. In C. Mattingly & M. H. Fleming, *Clinical reasoning: Forms of inquiry in therapeutic practice* (pp. 3–21). Philadelphia: F. A. Davis.

Fleming, M. H., & Mattingly, C. (2000). Action and narrative: Two dynamics of clinical reasoning. In J. Higgs & M. Jones (Eds.), *Clinical reasoning in the health professions* (2nd ed.), (pp. 54–61). Oxford: Butterworth-Heinemann.

Fondiller, E., Rosage, L. J., & Neuhaus, B. E. (1990). Values influencing clinical reasoning in occupational therapy: An exploratory study. *Occupational Therapy Journal of Research, 10*(1), 41–55.

Fortune, T., & Ryan, S. (1996). Applying clinical reasoning: A caseload management system for community occupational therapists. *British Journal of Occupational Therapy, 59*(5), 207–211.

Frank, G. (1996). Life histories in occupational therapy clinical practice. *American Journal of Occupational Therapy, 50*(4), 251–264.

Frank, J. D. (1958). The therapeutic use of self. *American Journal of Occupational Therapy, 12*(4), 215–225.

Frankl, V. E. (1963). *Man's search for meaning: An introduction to logotherapy.* New York: Washington Square Press.

Frankl, V. E. (1986). *Doctor and the soul: From psychotherapy to logotherapy.* New York: Vintage Books.

Freud, S. (1949). *An outline of psycho-analysis* (J. Strachey, Trans. and Ed.). New York: W. W. Norton.

Freud, S. (1960a). *The ego and the id.* (J. Riviere, Trans.; J. Strachey, Ed.). New York: W.W. Norton.

Freud, S. (1960b). *The psychopathology of everyday life* (A. Tyson, Trans.; J. Strachey, Ed.). New York: W. W. Norton.

Friedman, M. (1965). Introductory essay. In M. Buber, *The knowledge of man* (pp. 11–58). New York: Harper and Row.

Fromm, E. (1992). *Art of being.* New York: Continuum.

Fromm, E. (1994). *Art of listening.* New York: Continuum.

Gazda, G. M., Walters, R. P., & Childers, W. C. (1975). *Human relations development: A manual for health sciences.* Boston: Allyn and Bacon.

Gillette, N., & Mattingly, C. (1987). Clinical reasoning in occupational therapy. *American Journal of Occupational Therapy, 41*(6), 399–400.

Gitlin, L. N., Corcoran, M. C., & Leinmiller-Eckhardt, S. (1995). Understanding the family perspective: An ethnographic framework for providing occupational therapy in the home. *American Journal of Occupational Therapy, 49,* 802–809.

Hagedorn, R. (1995). Therapeutic use of self. In *Occupational therapy: Perspectives and processes* (pp. 259–267.). London: Churchill Livingston.

Hall, L., Robertson, W., Turner, M. A. (1992). Clinical reasoning process for service provision in the public school. *American Journal of Occupational Therapy, 46*(10), 927–936.

Hallin, M., & Sviden, G. (1995). On expert occupational therapists' reflection-on-practice. *Scandinavian Journal of Occupational Therapy, 2*(20), 69–75.

Hasselkus, B. R. (1989). The meaning of daily activity in family caregiving for the elderly. *American Journal of Occupational Therapy, 43*(10), 649–656.

Hasselkus, B. R. (1994). Professionals and informal caregivers: The therapeutic alliance. In B. Bonder & M. Wagner (Eds.), *Functional performance in older adults* (pp. 339–351). Philadelphia: F. A. Davis.

Hasselkus, B. R., & Dickie, V. (1990). Themes of meaning: Occupational therapists' perspectives on practice. *Occupational Therapy Journal of Research, 10*, 195–207.

Higgs, J., & Jones, M. (1995). *Clinical reasoning in the health professions.* Oxford: Butterworth-Heinemann.

Higgs, J., & Jones, M. (2000). Clinical reasoning in the health professions. In J. Higgs & M. Jones (Eds.), *Clinical reasoning in the health professions* (2nd ed.) (pp. 3–14). Oxford: Butterworth-Heinemann.

Higgs, J., & Titchen, A. (2000). Knowledge and reasoning. In J. Higgs & M. Jones (Eds.), *Clinical reasoning in the health professions* (2nd ed.) (pp. 23–32). Oxford: Butterworth-Heinemann.

Hooper, B. (1997). The relationship between pretheoretical assumptions and clinical reasoning. *American Journal of Occupational Therapy, 51*(5), 328–338.

Horney, K. (1937). *The neurotic personality of our time.* New York: W. W. Norton.

Horney, K. (1939). *New ways in psychoanalysis.* New York: W. W. Norton.

Horney, K. (1945). *Our inner conflicts: A constructive theory of neurosis.* New York: W. W. Norton.

Horney, K. (1950). *Neurosis and human growth: The struggle toward self-realization.* New York: W. W. Norton.

Howe, M. C., & Schwartzberg, S. L. (1995). *A functional approach to group work in occupational therapy* (2nd ed.). Philadelphia: J. B. Lippincott.

Howe, M. C., & Schwartzberg, S. L. (2001). *A functional approach to group work in occupational therapy* (3rd ed.). Philadelphia: Lippincott Williams & Wilkins.

Jones, J. (1991). Therapeutic use of metaphor. *Nursing Standard, 6*(11), 30–32.

Jordan, J. V. (1997). Relational development through mutual empathy. In A. C. Bohart and L. S. Greenberg (Eds.), *Empathy reconsidered: New directions in psychotherapy* (pp. 343–351). Washington, DC: American Psychological Association.

Jordan, J., Kaplan, A., Miller, J. B., Stiver, I., & Surrey, J. (1991). *Women's growth in connection.* New York: Guilford Press.

Kautzmann, L. N. (1993). Linking patient and family stories to caregivers' use of clinical reasoning. *American Journal of Occupational Therapy, 47*(2), 169–173.

Kielhofner, G. (1983). *Health through occupation: Theory and practice in occupational therapy.* Philadelphia: F. A. Davis.

Kielhofner, G. (1985). *A model of human occupation: Theory and application.* Baltimore: Williams and Wilkins.

Kielhofner, G. (1995). *A model of human occupation: Theory and application* (2nd ed.). Baltimore: Williams and Wilkins.

Kielhofner, G. (1997). *Conceptual foundations of occupational therapy* (2nd ed.). Philadelphia: F. A. Davis.

Kielhofner, G., & Nicol, M. (1989). The model of human occupation: A developing conceptual tool for clinicians. *British Journal of Occupational Therapy, 52*(6), 210–214.

King, M., Novik, L., & Citrenbaum, C. (1983). *Irresistible communication: Creative skills for the health professional.* Philadelphia: W. B. Saunders.

Langthaler, M. (1990). *The components of therapeutic relationship in occupational therapy.* Unpublished master's thesis, Tufts University, Medford, MA.

Law, M. (Ed.). (1998). *Client-centered occupational therapy.* Thorofare, NJ: Slack.

Lawlor, M. C., & Mattingly, C. (1998). The complexities of family-centered care. *American Journal of Occupational Therapy, 52*(4), 259–267.

Linehan, M. M. (1997). Validation and psychotherapy. In A. C. Bohart and L. S. Greenberg (Eds.), *Empathy reconsidered: New directions in psychotherapy* (pp. 353–392). Washington, DC: American Psychological Association.

Lowenstein, A., & Schwartzberg, S. L. (1999). A support group for head-injured individuals: Stories from the peer leader and facilitator. In S. Ryan, and E. McKay, *Thinking and reasoning in therapy: Narratives from practice* (pp. 94–106). Cheltenham, England: Stanley Thornes.

MacKinnon, J. L., & Rae, N. M. (1996). Fostering geriatric interdisciplinary collaboration through academic education. *Physical and Occupational Therapy in Geriatrics, 14*(3), 41–49.

MacRae, A., & Cara, E. (1998). The occupational therapy process in mental health. In A. MacRae and E. Cara (Eds.), *Psychosocial occupational therapy: A clinical practice* (pp. 3–31). Albany, NY: Delmar.

Mahler, M. S. (1968). *On human symbiosis and the vicissitudes of individuation.* New York: International Universities Press.

Mahler, M. S., Pine, F., & Bergman, A. (1975). *The psychological birth of the human infant: Symbiosis and individuation.* New York: Basic Books.

Maslow, A. H. (1968). *Toward a psychology of being* (2nd ed.). Princeton, NJ: D. Van Nostrand.

Maslow, A. H. (1987). *Motivation and personality* (3rd ed.). New York: Harper and Row. (Originally published in 1954)

Mattingly, C. (1991a). What is clinical reasoning? *American Journal of Occupational Therapy, 45,* 979–986.

Mattingly, C. (1991b). The narrative nature of clinical reasoning. *American Journal of Occupational Therapy, 45,* 998–1005.

Mattingly, C. (1998). *Healing dramas and clinical plots: The narrative structure of experience.* Cambridge: Cambridge University Press.

Mattingly, C., & Beer, D. W. (1995). School diversity: Strategies for bridging children's cultural world. In AOTA, *Conference Abstracts and Resources 1995* (pp. 29–30). Bethesda, MD: American Occupational Therapy Association.

Mattingly, C., & Fleming, M. H. (1994). Interactive reasoning: Collaborating with the person. In C. Mattingly and M. H. Fleming, *Clinical reasoning: Forms of inquiry in a therapeutic practice* (pp. 178–196). Philadelphia: F. A. Davis.

Mattingly, C., & Gillette, N. (1991). Anthropology, occupational therapy, and action research. *American Journal of Occupational Therapy, 45*(11), 972–978.

McKay, E. A., & Ryan, S. (1995). Clinical reasoning through story telling: Examining a student's case story on a fieldwork placement. *British Journal of Occupational Therapy, 58*(6), 234–238.

McLeod, J., & Balamoutsou, S. (1996). Representing narrative process in therapy: Qualitative analysis of a single case. *Counselling Psychology Quarterly, 9*(1), 61–76.

Medhurst, A., & Ryan, S. (1996a). Clinical reasoning in local authority paediatric occupational therapy: Planning a major adaptation for the child with a degenerative condition, Part 1. *British Journal of Occupational Therapy, 59*(5), 203–206.

Medhurst, A., & Ryan, S. (1996b). Clinical reasoning in local authority paediatric occupational therapy: Planning a major adaptation for the child with a degenerative condition, Part 2. *British Journal of Occupational Therapy, 59*(6), 269–272.

Mew, M. M., & Fossey, E. (1996). Client-centred aspects of clinical reasoning during initial assessment using the Canadian Occupational Performance Measure. *Australian Occupational Therapy Journal, 43,* 155–166.

Mosey, A. C. (1968). Recapitulation of ontogenesis: A theory for practice of occupational therapy. *American Journal of Occupational Therapy, 22*(5), 426–432.

Mosey, A. C. (1970). The concept and use of developmental groups. *American Journal of Occupational Therapy, 24*(4), 272–275.

Mosey, A. C. (1973). *Activities therapy.* New York: Raven Press.

Mosey, A. C. (1981). *Occupational therapy: Configuration of a profession.* New York: Raven Press.

Mostert, E., & Zacharkiewicz, A., & Fossey, E. (1996). Claiming the illness experience: Using narrative to enhance theoretical understanding (in process). *Australian Occupational Therapy Journal, 43*(3/4), 125–132.

Munroe, H. (1996). Clinical reasoning in community occupational therapy. *British Journal of Occupational Therapy, 59*(5), 196–202.

Navarra, T., Lipkowitz, M. A., & Navarra, J. G. (1990). *Therapeutic communication: A guide to effective interpersonal skills for health care professionals.* Thorofare, NJ: Slack.

Neistadt, M. E. (1987). Classroom as clinic: A model for teaching clinical reasoning in occupational therapy education. *American Journal of Occupational Therapy, 41*(10), 631–637.

Neistadt, M. E. (1992). The classroom as clinic: Applications for a method of teaching clinical reasoning. *American Journal of Occupational Therapy, 46*(9), 814–819.

Neistadt, M. E. (1996). Teaching strategies for the development of clinical reasoning. *American Journal of Occupational Therapy, 50*(8), 676–684.

Neistadt, M. E. (1998). Teaching clinical reasoning as a thinking frame. *American Journal of Occupational Therapy, 52*(3), 221–229.

Neistadt, M. E., & Atkins, A. (1996). Analysis of the orthopedic content in an occupational therapy curriculum from a clinical reasoning perspective. *American Journal of Occupational Therapy, 50*(8), 669–675.

Neistadt, M. E., Wight, J., & Mulligan, S. E. (1998). Clinical reasoning case studies as teaching tools. *American Journal of Occupational Therapy, 52*(2), 125–132.

Nitsun, M. (1996). *The anti-group: Destructive forces in the group and their creative potential.* New York: Routledge.

Norrby, E., & Bellner, A. (1995). The helping encounter: Occupational therapists' perception of therapeutic relationships. *Scandinavian Journal of Caring Science, 9,* 41–46.

Patel, V. L., & Arocha, J. F. (2000). Methods in the study of clinical reasoning. In J. Higgs & M. Jones (Eds.), *Clinical reasoning in the health professions* (2nd ed.) (pp. 78–91). Oxford: Butterworth-Heinemann.

Peloquin, S. (1988). Linking purpose to procedure during interactions with patients. *American Journal of Occupational Therapy, 42,* 775–781.

Peloquin, S. (1990). The patient-therapist relationship in occupational therapy: Understanding visions and images. *American Journal of Occupational Therapy, 44,* 13–21.

Peloquin, S. (1993). The depersonalization of patients: A profile gleaned from narratives. *American Journal of Occupational Therapy, 47*(9), 830–837.

Peloquin, S. M. (1995). The fullness of empathy: Reflections and illustrations. *American Journal of Occupational Therapy, 49*(1), 24–31.

Peloquin, S. M. (1998). The therapeutic relationship. In M. E. Neistadt and E. B. Crepeau (Eds.), *Willard and Spackman's occupational therapy* (9th ed.) (pp. 105–119). Philadelphia: J. B. Lippincott.

Peloquin, S. M., & Davidson, D. A. (1993). Interpersonal skills for practice: An elective course. *American Journal of Occupational Therapy, 47*(3), 260–264.

Perrin, T., & May, H. (2000). *Wellbeing in dementia: An occupational approach for therapists and carers.* London: Churchill Livingstone.

Price-Lackey, P., & Cashman, J. (1996). Jenny's story: Reinventing oneself through occupation and narrative configuration. *American Journal of Occupational Therapy, 50*(4), 306–314.

Purtilo, R. (1984). *Health professional/patient interaction* (3rd ed.). Philadelphia: W. B. Saunders.

Purtilo, R., & Haddad, A. (1996). *Health professional and patient interaction* (5th ed.). Philadelphia: W. B. Saunders.

Reilly, M. (1966). A psychiatric occupational therapy program as a teaching model. *American Journal of Occupational Therapy, 20*(2), 61–67.

Reilly, M. (1969). The education process. *American Journal of Occupational Therapy, 23*(4), 299–307.

Roberts, A. E. (1996). Approaches to reasoning in occupational therapy: A critical exploration. *British Journal of Occupational Therapy, 59*(5), 233–236.

Robertson, L. (1999). Assessing Mabel at home: A complex problem-solving process. In S. Ryan, and E. McKay (Eds.), *Thinking and reasoning in therapy: Narratives from practice* (pp. 19–30). Cheltenham, England: Stanley Thornes.

Robertson, L. J. (1996). Clinical reasoning, part 1: The nature of problem solving, a literature review. *British Journal of Occupational Therapy, 59*(4), 178–182.

Rogers, C. R. (1940/1992). The processes of therapy. *Journal of Consulting and Clinical Psychology, 60*(2), 163–164. (Originally published in 1940 in *Journal of Consulting Psychology, 4,* 161–164)

Rogers, C. R. (1957/1992). The necessary and sufficient conditions of therapeutic personality change. *Journal of Consulting Psychology, 60*(6), 827–832. (Originally published in 1957 in *Journal of Consulting Psychology, 21,* 95–103)

Rogers, C. R. (1959). A theory of therapy, personality and interpersonal relationships, as developed in the client-centered framework. In S. Koch (Ed.), *Psychology: A study of a science: Vol. 3. Formulation of the person and the social context* (pp. 184–256). New York: McGraw-Hill.

Rogers, C. R. (1962). *On becoming a person.* Boston: Houghton Mifflin.

Rogers, C. R. (1965). *Client-centered therapy: Its current practice, implications and theory.* Boston: Houghton Mifflin.

Rogers, J. C., & Holm, M. B. (1991). Occupational therapy diagnostic reasoning: A component of clinical reasoning. *American Journal of Occupational Therapy, 45*(11), 1045–1053.

Rogers, J. C., & Masagatani, G. (1982). Clinical reasoning of occupational therapists during initial assessment of physically disabled patients. *Occupational Therapy Journal of Research, 2*(4), 195–219.

Rosa, S. A., & Hasselkus, B. R. (1996). Connecting with patients: The personal experience of professional helping. *Occupational Therapy Journal of Research, 16*(4), 245–260.

Royeen, C. B. (1995). A problem-based learning curriculum for occupational therapy education. *American Journal of Occupational Therapy, 49*(4), 338–346.

Ryan, S. (1999). Why narratives? In S. Ryan & E. McKay (Eds.), *Thinking and reasoning in therapy: Narratives from practice* (pp. 1–15). Cheltenham, England: Stanley Thornes.

Ryan, S., & McKay, E. (Eds.). (1999). *Thinking and reasoning in therapy: Narratives from practice.* Cheltenham, England: Stanley Thornes.

Schell, B. A. (1998). Clinical reasoning: The basis of practice. In M. E. Neistadt and E. B. Crepeau (Eds.), *Willard and Spackman's occupational therapy* (9th ed.) (pp. 90–100). Philadephia: J. B. Lippincott.

Schell, B. A., & Cervero, R. M. (1993). Clinical reasoning in occupational therapy: An integrative review. *American Journal of Occupational Therapy, 47,* 605–610.

Schell, B. A., & Cervero, R. M. (1995). The role of practice context in clinical reasoning. *American Occupational Therapy Association conference abstracts and resources 1995,* pp. 51–52. Bethesda, MD: American Occupational Therapy Association.

Schwartz, K. B. (1991). Clinical reasoning and new ideas on intelligence: Implications for teaching and learning. *American Journal of Occupational Therapy, 45*(11), 1033–1037.

Schwartzberg, S. L. (1993). Chapter 9: Tools of Practice, Section 1, Therapeutic use of self (pp. 269–274), and Section 2, Group process (pp. 275–280). In H. L. Hopkins, and H. D. Smith (Eds.), *Willard and Spackman's occupational therapy* (8th ed.). Philadelphia: J. B. Lippincott.

Schwartzberg, S. L. (1999). The use of groups in the rehabilitation of persons with head injury: Reasoning skills used by the group facilitator. In C. Unsworth, *Cognitive and perceptual dysfunction: A clinical reasoning approach to evaluation and intervention* (pp. 455–471). Philadelphia: F. A. Davis.

Sharrott, G. W. (1983). Occupational therapy's role in the client's creation and affirmation of meaning. In G. Kielhofner, *Health through occupation: Theory and practice in occupational therapy.* Philadelphia: F. A. Davis.

Slater, D. Y., & Cohn, E. S. (1991). Staff development through analysis of practice. *American Journal of Occupational Therapy, 45*(11), 1038–1044.

Spencer, J., Davidson, H., & White, V. (1997). Helping clients develop hopes for the future. *American Journal of Occupational Therapy, 51*(3),191–198.

Sullivan, H. S. (1953). *The interpersonal theory of psychiatry.* New York: W. W. Norton.

Sullivan, H. S. (1954). *The psychiatric interview.* New York: W. W. Norton.

Sviden, G., & Hallin, M. (1999). Differences in clinical reasoning between occupational therapists working in rheumatology and neurology. *Scandinavian Journal of Occupational Therapy, 6*(2), 63–69.

Sviden, G., & Saljo, R. (1993). Perceiving patients and their nonverbal reactions. *American Journal of Occupational Therapy, 47,* 491–497.

Tickle-Degnen, L. (2000). Evidence-based practice forum: Gathering current research evidence to enhance clinical reasoning. *American Journal of Occupational Therapy, 54*(1), 102–105.

Tomlin, G., & Stone, R. (1997). Computer networks and simulations to support patient care. *American Occupational Therapy Association Conference Abstracts and Resources 1991,* pp. 31–32. Bethesda, MD: American Occupational Therapy Association.

Toth-Cohen, S. (2000). Role perceptions of occupational therapists providing support and education for caregivers of persons with dementia. *American Journal of Occupational Therapy, 54*(5), 509–515.

Tryssenaar, J. (1995). Interactive journals: An educational strategy to promote reflection. *American Journal of Occupational Therapy, 49*(7), 695–702.

Unsworth, C. (1999). *Cognitive and perceptual dysfunction: A clinical reasoning approach to evaluation and intervention.* Philadelphia: F. A. Davis.

VanLeit, B. (1995). Using the case method to develop clinical reasoning skills in problem-based learning. *American Journal of Occupational Therapy, 49*(4) 349–353.

White, R. W. (1959). Motivation reconsidered: The concept of competence. *American Psychological Review, 66,* 297–333.

White, R. W. (1971). The urge toward competence. *American Journal of Occupational Therapy, 25*(6), 271–274.

Winnicott, D. W. (1965). *The family and individual development.* London: Tavistock Publications.

Winnicott, D. W. (1971). *Playing and reality.* New York: Basic Books.

Winnicott, D. W. (1987). *Holding and interpretation: Fragment of an analysis.* New York: Grove Press.

Winnicott, D. W. (1988). *Human nature.* New York: Schocken Books.

Yerxa, E. (1967). 1966 Eleanor Clarke Slagle lecture, Authentic occupational therapy. *American Journal of Occupational Therapy, 21*(1), 1–9.

Yuen, H. K., & Yau, M. K. (1999). Cross-cultural awareness and occupational therapy education. *Occupational Therapy International, 6*(1), 24–34.

INDEX